2nd Edition

Student Practice Supervision & Assessment

A Guide for NMC Nurses & Midwives

Jo Lidster
Susan Wakefield

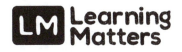

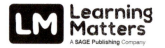

Learning Matters
A SAGE Publishing Company
1 Oliver's Yard
55 City Road
London EC1Y 1SP

SAGE Publications Inc.
2455 Teller Road
Thousand Oaks, California 91320

SAGE Publications India Pvt Ltd
B 1/I 1 Mohan Cooperative Industrial Area
Mathura Road
New Delhi 110 044

SAGE Publications Asia-Pacific Pte Ltd
3 Church Street
#10-04 Samsung Hub
Singapore 049483

First edition published 2019
Second edition 2022

Editor: Laura Walmsley
Development editor: Sarah Turpie
Senior project editor: Chris Marke
Project management: River Editorial
Cover design: Wendy Scott
Typeset by: C&M Digitals (P) Ltd, Chennai, India

Library of Congress Control Number: 2021942043

British Library Cataloguing in Publication Data

A catalogue record for this book is available from the British Library

ISBN 978-1-5297-3391-4
ISBN 978-1-5297-3390-7 (pbk)

Student Practice Supervision & Assessment

Contents

About the authors

Jo Lidster is the Deputy Head of the Department of Nursing and Midwifery at Sheffield Hallam University. Jo leads on postgraduate and continuing professional development provision for the department as well as on placement learning initiatives. This involves working closely with practice learning partners and other stakeholders to develop a quality learning experience. Jo is an adult nurse and prior to working in education she worked in and managed several acute and critical care areas. She teaches a range of undergraduate and postgraduate students on topics including research methods and evidence-based practice, healthcare education, supervision and assessment. Jo's research interests include student support and supervision models, as well as the use of technology in learning.

Susan Wakefield is the Head of Nursing and Midwifery at Sheffield Hallam University. She is responsible for educational and practice provision for all the undergraduate and postgraduate students who study with the department. She works closely with the wider university leadership team, senior practice learning partners and other stakeholders to ensure provision is high quality. During her time in higher education, Susan has worked at department, college and university level in a number of roles. She is a mental health nurse and has had a range of roles in clinical practice including research nurse, care pathways co-ordinator and community mental health nurse. She teaches research methods and evidence-based practice and supervises postgraduate students. Susan's research interests include the use of technology to support behaviour change.

About this book

This book is a handbook; an easy-to-use guide for Nursing and Midwifery Council (NMC) registrants who are involved in supervising and assessing nursing and midwifery students in practice settings. You may be a newly qualified nurse or midwife or possibly have a wealth of experience in supervising and assessing students. You may be at the start of your supervisor journey or you may have already completed an NMC-approved mentor-preparation programme. Either way, we think you will find this book useful. For those of you with less experience of practice supervising and assessing students, it includes information and activities to enhance your understanding. This includes educational theories and evidence-based models to develop your practice supervisor and assessor attributes and skills. For the reader who is more experienced, the book clearly describes the NMC standards and roles, and suggests how these can be applied to your developing practice. We intend that it will also stretch your understanding and enhance your practice regardless of your existing knowledge and experience. As a result, we hope the book enables you to provide the best learning experience for students, while protecting the public through robust assessment processes.

It is not intended that you read the book from start to finish, or necessarily cover to cover. However, we suggest you do start with Chapter 1, which is an introduction, and then *dip into* the rest of the book as you see fit. If you are new to working with students, you may wish to read each chapter in order. If you are an established supervisor or assessor, you may find it more helpful to focus on specific sections or chapters. The contents page and chapter aims at the beginning of each chapter will help you choose which are most relevant to you.

This book is closely mapped to the new NMC *Standards Framework for Nursing and Midwifery Education* published in 2018. These standards have replaced the NMC *Standards to Support Learning and Assessment in Practice* (2008). The book aims to bring the standards to life and help you apply them in your professional practice. We have mapped the content from each chapter against *Part 1: Standards Framework for Nursing and Midwifery Education* (NMC, 2018d) so you can clearly identify how the chapters relate to these. We have also mapped each chapter's content to relevant professional standards from the Code (NMC, 2015). We have done this to help you recognise how the two are interlinked, as well as to support your NMC revalidation where you are required to map your learning against the Code.

Why this book?

We intend for this to be used as a handbook, containing the most important information about student supervision and assessment in a straightforward and accessible way. We hope you find this easy to refer to and helpful to you in your role.

It is not designed to be a theoretical book focusing heavily on the evidence base for educational approaches. However, we do refer to educational and interpersonal theories and models where relevant. We use these for you to consider how they might help you understand your role and develop your attributes and skills. It is a highly applied book, and we have referred to relevant theories and evidence in a way that complements the NMC standards. There are a number of scenarios and activities; these are included to develop your knowledge and skills as well as to help you apply the standards. We hope you view this book as a critical friend – something you can refer to and receive guidance from to boost your skills and confidence.

Book structure

The book is largely structured around the NMC *Standards for Student Supervision and Assessment* (2018). The chapter titles of Chapters 2–5 and 7 directly reflect the sections of these standards. The additional chapters complement the standards and add some further perspectives when supervising and assessing students.

Chapter 1: Introduction to supervision and assessment in practice. This chapter describes the standards and what the responsibilities are for those undertaking the new roles. It provides a brief overview of the previous standards as the terms used in these will be something you will encounter on a regular basis. We explore the importance of reflective practice in developing as a supervisor and assessor, as well as for your NMC revalidation. We then look at the wider team who are involved in supporting students and student learning, and how these roles interface.

Chapter 2: Learning culture. This chapter aims to help you understand the best learning environment for students to thrive in and be able to meet all the requirements of their placement and educational programme. After reading the chapter and completing the activities, you should have a better understanding of the features of a good learning environment. It will help you develop your understanding not only of your role in developing a great learning culture but also of the role of colleagues and partners in making this happen. We also consider how to support students with diverse needs and those who may have learning contracts and require reasonable adjustments.

Chapter 3: Educational governance and quality. The governance and quality processes that need to be implemented to ensure the safe and effective delivery of student learning and assessment are covered in this chapter. These processes and decisions need to be robust to protect the public. We include which processes need to be in place to recruit students onto programmes and ensure safe practice learning environments. We also describe the governance involved in supporting students who are struggling or indeed those who fail to achieve their placement learning outcomes. There is a section on students' *fitness to practise* issues and how to manage this. Finally, we consider how to support students who escalate concerns about poor practice which they have observed while on placement.

Chapter 4: Student empowerment. This chapter summarises the evidence base in relation to how people learn, including learning theories and styles. Understanding how we learn can empower us to take control of our own learning requirements and become self-directed. We suggest how you might adapt your teaching and learning approaches to accommodate different learning styles and preferences, thereby creating the best environment for a range of students. The chapter then considers other learning and teaching approaches you can adopt such as peer learning and interprofessional learning. We conclude by examining how generational differences may impact on learning and how you, as supervisor and/or assessor, can facilitate learning opportunities that will appeal to a range of generations.

Chapter 5: Supervisors, assessors and educators. The skills and attributes required of supervisors and assessors and how you can develop these are the focus of this chapter. We also introduce the benefits that can be gained by working collaboratively to support student practice learning. Using learning objectives to maximise learning opportunities is examined, with the aim of supporting your students to be able to recognise their own learning needs. We then outline common teaching methods that you can use in your role and the advantages and disadvantages of these methods. This will provide you with a repertoire of teaching methods to draw upon to meet your students' learning needs wherever possible.

Chapter 6: Coaching models and approaches. This chapter introduces coaching models and approaches. It builds upon Chapters 4 and 5 to present coaching as an approach to student support that is both facilitative and encourages students to actively participate in their own learning. The focus of this chapter is on applying a coaching approach to student practice supervision and assessment, and scenarios are used to apply models to situations you may already be familiar with. Organisational models of coaching used to support student practice supervision and assessment are highlighted, and the chapter concludes with the wider uses of coaching for your own career.

Chapter 7: Curricula and assessment. This chapter will help you recognise your role in understanding and engaging with your students' curricula and develop your understanding of assessment and competence. Understanding assessment approaches and assessment theory is essential in helping us to make robust decisions. We will help you to develop your understanding of different methods that can be used to assess student competence and the benefits of using assessment approaches that involve a range of colleagues. We then examine the importance of feedback, including its purpose, the benefits of high-quality feedback on learning and the principles of good feedback. The chapter also covers how to best support students in difficulty, who for whatever reason are struggling to progress. We then move on to assessments and consider how you can use established processes to manage failing students, as well as the importance of getting support for yourself if you find yourself in this complex situation.

Chapter 8: Developing yourself as a supervisor and/or assessor. The focus of this chapter is on you and your developing role as a supervisor and/or assessor. We begin by looking at developing your wellbeing and resilience and the importance of these in your role. We then look at some common and useful techniques for you to develop both your own and your students' resilience. Building on earlier chapters, we consider how useful resilience is when you are working with students in difficulty or when things *go wrong*. The final section of the chapter offers you the opportunity to review your continuing professional development needs. We also suggest how to use your newly acquired knowledge and skills to further develop both your colleagues and your profession.

Learning features

Learning from reading text is not always easy. Therefore, to provide variety and to assist in applying the learning and NMC standards to practice, this book contains activities, case studies, scenarios, further reading, useful websites and other materials to enable you to participate in your own learning. You will need to develop your own study skills and *learn how to learn* to get the best from the material. The book cannot provide all the answers, but provides a framework for your learning.

Some activities ask you to reflect on aspects of practice, or your experience of it, or the people or situations you encounter. *Reflection* is an essential skill in nursing and midwifery, and it helps you to understand the world around you and often to identify how things might improve. Other activities will help you develop key skills such as your ability to *think critically* about a topic in order to challenge perceived wisdom, and to be able to *make decisions* using that evidence in situations that are often difficult and time-pressured. Communication and working as part of a team are core to all nursing and midwifery practice, and some activities will ask you to carry out *teamwork activities*. Finally, as a registered nurse or midwife you will be expected to *lead and manage*, and so some activities focus on helping you build confidence in doing this.

All the activities require you to take a break from reading the text, think through the issues presented and carry out some independent study, possibly using the internet. Where appropriate, there are sample answers presented at the end of each chapter, and these will help you to understand more fully your own reflections and independent study.

You might want to think about completing these activities as part of your NMC revalidation. After completing the activity, write it up using the NMC revalidation forms and templates (**http://revalidation.nmc.org.uk/welcome-to-revalidation**) and keep it safe so you can use it when it is time for you to revalidate.

This book also contains a Glossary on page 179 to assist you with unfamiliar terms. Glossary terms are in bold in the first instance that they appear.

We do hope you enjoy this book and that it helps you on your exciting journey as a practice supervisor and/or practice assessor!

Chapter 1

Introduction to supervision and assessment in practice

Standards Framework for Nursing and Midwifery Education (NMC, 2018b)

This chapter will address all of the standards: 1: Learning culture, 2: Educational governance and quality, 3: Student empowerment, 4: Educators and assessors and 5: Curricula and assessment.

The Code: Professional Standards of Practice and Behaviour for Nurses and Midwives (NMC, 2015)

This chapter most closely aligns with the following professional standards.

Practise effectively

6.1 make sure that any information or advice given is evidence-based, including information relating to using any healthcare products or services.

6.2 maintain the knowledge and skills you need for safe and effective practice.

9 share your skills, knowledge and experience for the benefit of people receiving care and your colleagues (9.1–9.4).

Promote professionalism and trust

20 uphold the reputation of your profession at all times (20.1–20.10).

25.2 support any staff you may be responsible for to follow the Code at all times. They must have the knowledge, skills and competence for safe practice, and understand how to raise any concerns linked to any circumstances where the Code has been, or could be, broken.

> ## Chapter aims
>
> ....
>
> After reading this chapter you will be able to:
>
> - describe the key principles of the NMC (2018b) *Standards for Student Supervision and Assessment;*
> - describe the benefits of reflective practice to your role as practice supervisor/ practice assessor;
> - understand the roles of others involved in supporting students in practice;
> - describe some of the models used to support learners in practice.

Introduction

Think back to when you were a student. Remember how you felt on those first few hours or days in a new placement area. What helped to settle your nerves and develop your confidence? For many of us it was a mentor or supervisor: the person who welcomed us into their world and guided us through an often complex landscape. Those of us who have been fortunate enough to have an inspirational supervisor remember the impact they had on our practice. They act as an experienced guide leading us through unfamiliar terrain, working with us to reach our destination.

Student nurses place a high value on their practice experience and consider it one of the most important aspects of their pre-registration course. In addition, given that students spend 50 per cent of their time in practice, the relationship they have with their supervisor is central to their development.

Safe preparation of registrants, and others with caring roles, is critical to both patient safety and good patient outcomes. The time you invest in your role as supervisor or assessor, while not always recognised, will have a huge impact on the quality of today's and tomorrow's health professionals. The supervision and assessment of learners is highly valued in today's NHS and the Shape of Caring review highlighted its importance to patient care and safeguarding:

> *This complex role requires support and training. Going beyond teaching knowledge and skills, it involves displaying and modelling leadership attributes. The mentor [sic] must be conscious of students' individual needs and requirements and create an atmosphere conducive to learning. Positive role modelling and the opportunity for reflective practice are vital.*
>
> (Willis Commission, 2012, p33)

As a practice supervisor and/or practice assessor, you will develop both professionally and personally. Professionally, it might be the first step in a teaching career and helps with future career aspirations, as experienced practice supervisors are always valued by employers. Being a supervisor or assessor is a privileged position with the opportunity to impact hugely on student experience and, ultimately, patient care. Given this, we hope you see the importance of the role/s of practice supervisor/practice assessor you are about to embark on for both the current and future workforce.

This chapter will introduce you to the roles and responsibilities of the practice supervisor and practice assessor roles, as well as the NMC *Standards for Student Supervision and Assessment* (SSSA) (NMC, 2018b). In this chapter we meet Sylvie and Aleksandra to better understand how the standards apply to practice. You will have an opportunity to consider how reflective practice might enhance your skills as a supervisor/assessor. We then identify and describe 'the team around the student', who may be part of your organisation, or other organisations such as a university. The chapter concludes by introducing you to some models used to support learners in practice.

Scenario 1.1

Sylvie is an experienced registrant who works in a community team. She has been working with students as an NMC mentor and has previously undertaken an **NMC-approved** mentor-preparation programme. Working with students is one of her favourite parts of her job and she often finds herself organising learning resources and opportunities for the students within the team. Sylvie is now working with her managers and the link academic from her local university to implement the new SSSA within her organisation. She is keen to understand how her mentor experience and qualification will fit with the new practice supervisor and practice assessor roles. Sylvie is working with Aleksandra who has just started her first post with the community team. Aleksandra had an introduction as to how to support learners in practice in the final year of her pre-registration course. She also has personal experience of being supported as a student. Sylvie has been allocated as Aleksandra's preceptor* and will be supporting her to develop as a practice supervisor during the preceptorship period.

* A preceptor is an experienced registrant who provides support, for a given period, to new registrants joining the register to help with their transition.

This chapter's Scenario helps illustrate how influential the roles of practice supervisor and/or practice assessor are in today's healthcare environment. We can easily forget the range and longevity of a supervisor or assessor's scope of influence. Sylvie has supported many pre-registration students, who themselves have gone on to support many students. Each of those nurses has cared for hundreds of patients; therefore Sylvie's scope of influence is huge. The Scenario intends to highlight how valuable the roles of practice supervisor and practice assessor are in ensuring high-quality, compassionate care (Pritchard and Gidman, 2012).

In May 2018 the NMC overhauled its standards for supporting and assessing students as part of a large-scale review of the NMC *Education and Training Standards.* You may be familiar with the previous standards, and it is likely you will still hear terminology from the previous standards, especially the term 'mentor', but this has role now been replaced. However, in this book, we will refer to 'mentors' when we outline relevant literature or policy that pre-dates the introduction of the new NMC education and training standards. It is important to remember also that many practice colleagues, like Sylvie in the Scenario, will have been mentors, and are now working as practice supervisors and/or practice assessors.

The SSSA replaces the mentor role with two distinct roles: the practice supervisor and the practice assessor. The NMC states that the practice supervisor can be any registered health and social care professional who facilitates and supports students with their practice learning where appropriate. The SLAiP (NMC, 2008) standards required mentors to undertake an NMC-approved preparation course before individuals could take on this role. This often led to waiting lists for potential mentors wanting to access such a course and could then impact the potential mentor numbers in a placement area. The SSSA recognises that preparation for the supervisor and assessor role is best governed by the employing organisation, working in collaboration with the student's university. Concerns had been raised about the quality of mentorship and assessment of practice being variable in the old model. Also, there is potential for a lack of objectivity in the assessment of students whom mentors have become very familiar with, leading to students passing when perhaps they should have failed. This increases the risk of 'failing to fail', a phrase derived from Kathleen Duffy's (2003) seminal work, which is discussed further in Chapter 7.

The standards for education and training

The new standards for education and training have replaced the SLAiP (NMC, 2008) and are composed of three parts:

- Part 1: Standards Framework for Nursing and Midwifery Education;
- Part 2: Standards for Student Supervision and Assessment;
- Part 3: *Programme Standards* – for pre-registration nursing education and prescribing programmes.

It is Part 2, the *Standards for Student Supervision and Assessment*, that we will look at in more detail throughout this book, as these set out the "expectations for the learning, support and supervision of students in the practice environment" (NMC, 2018b, p3) and outline how students are assessed for both theory and practice. At the onset of the COVID-19 pandemic the NMC published a set of temporary standards relating to education. These were the emergency standards for nursing and midwifery education (2020) which were largely phased out after September 2020 and replaced by the

Recovery programme standards (NMC, 2021). As part of these emergency standards, it was expected that all students would receive support, supervision and assessments in line with the SSSA during this period. The NMC recognised that the SSSA had been quickly and uniformly adopted nationally and should stay. This has led to the SSSA being adopted much more quickly than some **Approved Educational Institutions (AEIs)** and practice areas had originally planned.

The SSSA now apply to all NMC-approved education programmes and, as such, they relate to all fields of nursing and midwifery and span both pre-registration and post-registration programmes. The SSSA retain the supernumerary status of students and states they "must be supported to learn without being counted as part of the staffing required for safe and effective care" (p4). There is also reference to the supernumerary status of apprentices studying an NMC-approved programme with an integrated apprenticeship route. In relation to these students, the standards state that "this includes practice placements within their place of employment; this does not apply when they are working in their substantive role" (p4).

The SSSA comprise three broad headings and ten sections. This book covers each of these areas in detail, but this next section presents an overview of the main areas to begin to familiarise you with the underpinning principles and requirements.

Effective practice learning – This focuses on providing safe and effective learning opportunities for student nurses and midwives when engaged in practice-based learning. There is a requirement for AEIs and practice learning partners to work together to ensure that all the standards for supervision and assessment of students are met. One way of facilitating this is by nominating an individual to be responsible for actively supporting students and addressing any concerns in practice areas. This is a requirement of the SSSA and individuals in this role may have a range of titles such as Learning Environment Manager or Practice Educator. In addition, students must be given the opportunity to learn from a range of people, including service users and other students. This emphasis on learning beyond the supervisor is welcomed and should open up opportunities to learn from a range of professionals.

Another requirement, which again moves away from over-reliance on the student–supervisor relationship, is that all NMC registrants must actively contribute to practice learning to ensure practice learning is everyone's business, not just those who have been allocated as a supervisor or assessor. Learning opportunities come in many shapes and sizes and can be facilitated by a range of people the student will encounter. Learning should be tailored to meet students' needs, for example considering the programme they are on, where they are in the programme and the proficiencies they need to meet during the placement. Students should be encouraged to work with practice colleagues to construct and evaluate these opportunities and experiences; not just for themselves but for others too. Evaluation of and feedback on learning is an underpinning principle of good educational practice and something all supervisors and assessors should seek out. These aspects of learning are discussed throughout this book.

Supervision of students – The new SSSA separate out the roles of practice supervisor and practice assessor. Previously these roles were combined into the one 'mentor' role. This separation is intended to increase objectivity and therefore lead to more robust assessment processes and decisions. According to the SSSA, practice supervisors may be an NMC registrant but may also be another type of registered health and social care professional (e.g. Health and Care Professions Council, General Pharmaceutical Council or General Medical Council). If they are an NMC registrant, they do not need to be on the same part of the register, or in the same field of nursing as the student they are supervising. However, they must support learning in line with their 'scope of practice' (this is explained in Table 1.1).

You may have heard colleagues being confused as to the role of the supervisor in assessing students. Supervisors may also be assessors (if they meet the criteria), but not involved in both the supervising and assessing of the same students (however, this was temporarily allowed as an exception during the period covered by the emergency standards for nursing and midwifery education). The roles are clearly separated, with differing responsibilities. However, a practice supervisor will contribute to the assessment of the students' achievement of proficiency. The practice supervisor will provide written and verbal feedback, based on a number of observations, discussions and simulation, etc. This must be considered by the practice assessor when making judgements about achievement of proficiencies and progression or completion. If the supervisor has concerns about a student's competence or **fitness to practice (FtP)**, they should raise this with the practice assessor and the academic colleague linking to the practice area from the student's AEI as soon as possible. There must be adequate opportunity to discuss these concerns and action plan as necessary.

Another change regarding the practice supervisor role is around the preparation for the role. Previously, all registrants supporting students on **NMC-approved programmes** needed to have completed an NMC-approved mentor-preparation programme. This is no longer the case for practice supervisors. The SSSA state supervisors must be given ongoing support to prepare, reflect and develop effective supervision to be able to contribute to student learning and assessment. In addition, they need to be knowledgeable of the programme the student they are supervising is undertaking and any proficiencies they are required to meet. It is also helpful if they understand the practice assessment document that needs to be completed. This means that your organisation will have its own preparation arrangements for the practice supervisor role designed collaboratively with the AEI. Activity 1.1 will help to explore this further.

Activity 1.1   Critical thinking

Earlier we met Aleksandra, a newly qualified registrant who requires preparation to become a practice supervisor in her clinical area. Aleksandra is a child field nurse working in a child and adolescent mental health community team. This is a popular and busy student placement area that accepts students from all fields of nursing, midwifery and also physiotherapy and occupational therapy. Aleksandra is interested to know which students she can supervise.

Given what you have learnt already about the SSSA:

- Can Aleksandra be a practice supervisor?
- If so, which students can she supervise?
- Would she be able to make assessment decisions about a student's achievement of proficiencies?

There is a model answer for this activity at the end of this chapter.

You will have noted from completing Activity 1.1 that Aleksandra would require preparation and support for the role of practice supervisor. The NMC (2018b) states the preparation should include opportunities for supervisors to:

- receive ongoing support to prepare, reflect and develop for effective supervision and contribution to student learning and assessment;
- have an understanding of the proficiencies and programme outcomes they are supporting students to achieve.

Practice assessors require different support and preparation for the role. Chapter 5 of this book explores the preparation requirements for these two roles in more detail.

Assessment of students and confirmation of proficiency – This section of the new standards focuses on the responsibilities of those colleagues who are assessing either academic or practice achievement. These roles are now more clearly defined and there is a requirement that the assessors maintain a greater distance from the student's day-to-day support, to increase the rigour of assessment decisions. The SSSA include the requirement for students to be assigned a new practice and academic assessors for each part of the programme. The academic assessor role is for academic staff in the student's AEI. The practice assessor can be a registered nurse, midwife or nursing associate, or in the case of prescribing programmes, any qualified prescriber. Their role is to assess a student's practice learning for a placement or a series of placements. The practice assessor works with the academic assessor to make recommendations for progression for the student they are assigned to. Usually for pre-registration undergraduate degree programmes, students would be allocated a different academic assessor and practice assessor for years (parts) 1, 2 and 3. These requirements in the SSSA aim to make all assessment decisions more robust and objective. This is through assessors not working too closely with students, so relationships do not cause bias, and through regular triangulation of theoretical and practical learning.

The criteria in relation to the students for whom a registrant can act as assessor are more prescriptive than those applied to the supervisor role. Examples of how the criteria might manifest in practice are modelled in Table 1.1.

Type of student	Type of assessor	Can they assess?
Nursing student – adult field	Registered nurse – adult field	Yes
Nursing student – mental health field	Registered nurse – child field, working in child and adolescent setting	Yes Assessor is a registered nurse with appropriate equivalent experience for the student's field of practice
Nursing student – child field	Registered nurse – mental health field, working in an older adult dementia assessment unit	No Although the registrant is a registered nurse and suitably prepared to carry out the assessor role, they are not child field and do not have the appropriate equivalent experience of working with children
Midwifery student	Registered midwife	Yes The practice and academic assessors must be registered midwives
Specialist community public health nursing student, post-registration	Specialist community public health nurse (school nursing) student working in a 0–19 service	Yes Registered specialist community public health nurse and appropriate equivalent experience of children and young people
Nursing student – learning disability field	Academic assessor is a registered nurse mental health field	No The academic does not have appropriate equivalent experience with learning disabilities
Non-medical prescribing student, post-registration	Practice assessor is general practitioner who is an experienced designated medical practitioner (DMP)	Yes Although not an NMC registrant, in the case of prescribing programmes the practice assessor must be any qualified prescriber who has been prepared for the role

Table 1.1 Applying the NMC assessor criteria

In addition to the criteria presented in Table 1.1, practice assessors must maintain "current knowledge and expertise" (NMC, 2018b, p9) for the proficiencies and programme outcomes they are assessing. The practice assessor must work with the academic assessor when recommending the student for progression to the next part of the programme. Let us apply some of these criteria to the characters from Scenario 1.1. Sylvie is an NMC registrant (mental health field) and she has previously completed an NMC-approved mentor-preparation course, therefore she is eligible to assess pre-registration students. However, she must have the appropriate equivalent experience for the student's field of practice. That may have been gained because of her own field of practice being the same as that of the student she is assessing, or this may be because of the experience she has gained through her professional experience.

Practice assessors must base their assessment decisions in part on direct observation of students and must not rely solely on feedback from others. However, they do need to collect feedback from others, including written and verbal feedback from supervisors as well as testimonies from patients and service users. By doing this, they can triangulate information from different sources to help them make more reliable and valid decisions. The NMC is clear that a registrant cannot perform the roles of practice assessor and practice supervisor with the same student, although they may be simultaneously supervising other students. This all adds to objectivity in the assessment process. Assessment issues are covered in more detail in Chapter 7 of this book.

Practice assessors also require preparation for the role. They may be new to assessing students or they may have previously successfully completed an NMC-approved mentor-preparation programme, but however experienced they are in supporting learners in practice, in order to meet the requirements of the practice assessor role they need to demonstrate the following:

- interpersonal communication skills;
- conducting objective and evidence-based assessment of students;
- providing constructive feedback to facilitate professional development of others;
- knowledge of the assessment process and their role in it.

So how can an NMC registrant achieve this? If you have previously completed an NMC-approved mentor course like Sylvie, then you meet the criteria above. For example, Sylvie will complete some transitional learning facilitated by her organisation and the linking academics from her student's AEI to prepare her for the role. However, if you have not, then you must be able to evidence the above; this may be through continuing professional development activities related to the above outcomes. This can be evidenced with an established practice assessor or your line manager during your appraisal. Alternatively, you may complete an 'assessor preparation'-style course delivered collaboratively by your organisation or local AEI. This might involve online learning resources, workbooks or workshops. The preparation courses will not be approved by the NMC, as there is no requirement for this under the new SSSA, but it should provide you with opportunities to explore assessment and related issues in more detail. In addition to the preparation for the roles, practice assessors and practice supervisors must have access to ongoing support and training for the role, demonstrate continuing professional development (which is a requirement of revalidation) and be familiar with programme proficiencies and outcomes of the programme on which the student they are assessing is enrolled.

Activity 1.2 Critical thinking

You have met Sylvie, who is an experienced registrant working in a community team. She has been working with students as an NMC mentor and has previously undertaken an NMC-approved mentor-preparation programme.

Given what you have learnt already about the SSSA (NMC, 2018b) and the SLAiP standards (NMC, 2008):

1. Can Sylvie be a practice supervisor?
2. Can Sylvie be a practice assessor?
3. What information from the Scenario informed your answers?

There is a model answer for this activity at the end of this chapter.

You might have an opportunity to shape how the new roles are embedded into practice, and we would encourage you to do so as the role of adequately prepared supervisors and assessors of clinical practice remains critical in facilitating the development of future generations of nurses and midwives.

Using reflective practice to enhance your efficacy as supervisor and assessor

Reflecting on your practice is an essential aspect of nursing and midwifery and a requirement for your revalidation with the NMC. There is widespread recognition of the value of reflection and reflective practice as it helps to develop practice and enhances our ability to learn from and through experiences. It also supports us to manage the psychological demands or the emotional burden of care delivery. Reflection is essential in helping us consider quality aspects of care and areas for improvement. It helps those supporting practice learning to be aware of their own knowledge, skills and beliefs about students; learning; teaching and assessment. Analysing and thinking about our supervision and assessment experiences is a natural opportunity to deepen our skills. Howatson-Jones (2016) offers a useful guide if you are interested in reading further about what reflection is, why it is so important and how to use it in your practice.

Reflective models can help guide us with our reflective practice. A simple reflective cycle is suggested by Gibbs (1988). It is iterative and cyclical, in that Gibbs suggests we learn by repeating our experiences. The model has six stages:

1. Description
2. Feelings

3. Evaluation

4. Analysis

5. Conclusion

6. Action plans

Gibbs' model is commonly favoured within the health professions as it is clear and precise. It allows for description, analysis and evaluation of an experience to help an individual make sense of experiences and practice. Reflecting on its own is not enough; you then have to put into practice the learning you have gained to ensure it informs your future practice (Gibbs, 1988). There are many models available to guide reflection, and Gibbs' model is just one of those. As with any model, choose one that you find fits your particular style. Using models can help us master reflective practice and ensure we complete the whole cycle, as taking action is essential and reflective models prompt the individual to formulate an action plan. The further reading at the end of this chapter directs you to other reflective models if you are interested in finding out more. The centrality of reflection to the profession is exemplified in the revalidation requirements (NMC, 2017a). It is therefore unsurprising that being reflective as a practice supervisor and/or assessor is essential. Activity 1.3 offers an opportunity to critically think about reflecting on practice using a draft of a reflection form completed by Sylvie.

Activity 1.3   Critical thinking

Sylvie has been using Gibbs' (1988) model to reflect on a practice experience as part of her evidence for her upcoming **NMC revalidation**. The experience she has chosen is her involvement in developing a workbook for new practice supervisors in her organisation.

Please read through this draft of her reflection form.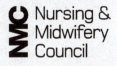

Reflective accounts form

You must use this form to record five written reflective accounts on your CPD and/or practice-related feedback and/or an event or experience in your practice and how this relates to the Code. Please fill in a page for each of your reflective accounts, making sure you do not include any information that might identify a specific patient, service user or colleague. Please refer to our guidance on preserving anonymity in the section on non-identifiable information in **How to revalidate with the NMC**.

(Continued)

(Continued)

Reflective account

What was the nature of the CPD activity and/or practice-related feedback and/or event or experience in your practice?

1. Description

I have been involved in developing a workbook to prepare colleagues to become practice supervisors for students. I have worked with others involved in supporting learners in practice, including community colleagues, managers and academics from the university. We also had students working with us to help us focus the content. We have had several meetings over the past six months and each taken responsibility to develop part of the workbook. The final workbook is now completed and has been signed off for use by the Trust management team. We are starting to use it and I have offered to evaluate the workbook over the next six months.

2. Feelings

I felt apprehensive at first when I read the new *Standards for Student Supervision and Assessment* (NMC, 2018b), as I could not imagine how we could 'lose' the mentor role. Mentoring is a big part of my professional identity and at first, I felt like I didn't want to give up this title. However, I was really pleased to be asked to take part in this work as I feel I have lots of experience from my previous mentor role which I was able to share and use for this workbook. I was also pleased to be part of a bigger team working on this and I enjoyed working with colleagues from different backgrounds.

What did you learn from the CPD activity and/or feedback and/or event or experience in your practice?

3. Evaluation

The new NMC (2018b) *Standards for Student Supervision and Assessment* have overhauled the previous standards and part of this has meant scrapping the mentor role. Instead, we are having two other roles to support learners. Organisations are free to decide who is best suited to supervise and assess students, as well as how they are prepared for these roles. The new standards should ensure students can be supervised at all times and by a range of registrants, rather than waiting for their designated mentor to become free.

This provides an opportunity for new staff to be practice supervisors and we need to be able to prepare them for this important role. We have developed a workbook that is easily accessible and can prepare any nursing, midwifery or allied health professional registrant who is interested in supporting students as a practice supervisor. Creating a workbook means we can support more staff in a timelier manner, rather than waiting for a place on a mentor course. It's important to be working **multi-professionally** on these sorts of initiatives, as that's how we are expecting our students to be able to work.

4. Analysis

We have had lots of colleagues inputting into this and worked in a collaborative way (Tasselli, 2015). I think this has really added to the quality of the workbook and hopefully has helped get others on board. Involving students as well has really helped to gain a focus on what's important for this role (Haraldseid et al., 2016). This has shaped my commitment to involve other colleagues, professions and students in the evaluation. I now feel less anxious about the changes and I have had time to really get to know the new standards (NMC, 2018) and think about what this means to practice.

How did you change or improve your practice as a result?

5. Conclusion

I have learnt that by creating a workbook we can support more staff in a timelier manner, rather than waiting for a place on a mentor course. It's important to be working multi-professionally on these sorts of initiatives, as that's how we are expecting our students to be able to work. I have also learnt that being involved in shaping and designing part of my organisation's implementation of the *Standards for Student Supervision and Assessment* (NMC, 2018b) has helped me better understand the standards and allay any anxieties I had. Although I might feel anxious about a change involving my 'mentor status', getting involved in the workbook has helped me to feel more in control about the changes and be more prepared for my new practice supervisor and practice assessor roles.

6. Action plans

How is this relevant to the Code?

Select one or more themes: Prioritise people – Practise effectively – Preserve safety – Promote professionalism and trust

Once you have read Sylvie's draft reflection:

1. Complete an action plan for Sylvie.
2. Look at the last section of the form and consider how this is relevant to the Code (NMC, 2015). You can read the Code online at **www.nmc.org. uk/standards/code/read-the-code-online**.

There is a model answer at the end of this chapter.

You may wish to share your reflections with your peers or manager during appraisal. Maybe you noted in Activity 1.3 that often actions from reflections involve sharing information with others. You could reflect upon an experience you have had in relation to supporting learners with a colleague who you know has been involved in supporting a particular student. This offers an opportunity to learn with and from others. As Sylvie will have found from her engagement with the SSSA and her involvement in developing the workbook, there is a wider team involved in supporting learners in practice.

The wider team involved in supporting the student

In today's world of **interprofessional learning** and working, and outcomes-focused patient care, a team approach to supporting student learning is essential. We have already learnt from the SSSA (NMC, 2018b) that other registered health professionals can act as practice supervisors for our students. We also know that the practice assessor is a separate role to supervisor, so already there are a minimum of two individuals supporting a student's learning in the clinical area. However, if we start to consider others from within our organisation whose role it is to support placement learning, along with those from the student's university, we start to see the scale of potential support available (see Figure 1.1). Studies have found that the best teams are diverse teams – diverse

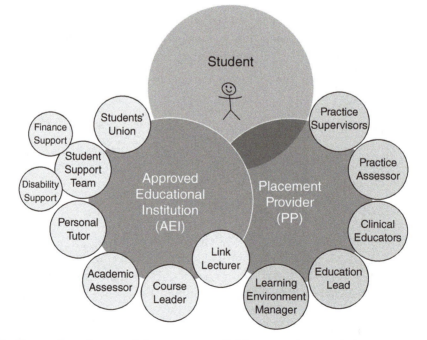

Figure 1.1   Examples of potential support available to students while on placement

in disciplines, professions, knowledge and abilities, as well as age, gender, background and life experiences, among others. Diversity hopefully represents different viewpoints and can help students make better decisions, find better solutions and produce better outcomes than individuals or homogeneous groups (Whitelock et al., 2015).

Figure 1.1 represents the triad arrangement of support involving the student, practice learning partners (PLPs) and AEIs. They all work collaboratively to support learning throughout the student's programme of study. You may already be aware of colleagues in your practice area whose role it is to support placement learning. Although these vary within organisations, they could include other practice supervisors and/or assessors, managers and education leads. There also exists a support network for the student from the student's AEI. These might include the student's personal tutor, designated student support staff and course leaders. Table 1.2 outlines common roles you might encounter in supporting students in the support they offer. Please note these roles will vary depending on the organisational requirements.

Roles	Definition and support offered
Practice supervisors	*Any registrant within the practice area who has been suitably prepared and supported to undertake the practice supervisor role.*
	Can support students by being a practice supervisor.
	Can help you to develop your supervision skills; support you with your development; provide a different viewpoint; and/or advise on student learning matters.
Practice assessors	*Any NMC registrant within the practice area who is an experienced supervisor and has been suitably prepared and supported to undertake the practice assessor role.*
	Can support students by being a practice assessor.
	Can help you to develop your supervisor/assessor skills; support you with your development; provide a different viewpoint; and/or advise on student learning matters.
Learning environment managers (LEMs)	*Usually a registrant based in each placement area who has a particular interest in supporting students in practice, and takes on additional related duties.*
	Can support students by directing them to learning resources and opportunities in the practice area.
	May allocate students to practice supervisors and/or practice assessors for the practice area. Will undertake the practice area educational audit and co-ordinates student evaluations for the area.
	Will have an overview of types of learners accessing your practice area, and the types of learning opportunities and proficiencies offered.
	Can help you to develop your skills; support you with your development; provide a different viewpoint; and/or advise on student learning matters.

(Continued)

Table 1.2   (Continued)

Roles	Definition and support offered
Clinical educators/practice educators/ professional development leads	*Usually expert clinical practitioners from a practice area with an educational focus, likely to have responsibility for training and development duties across a department or clinical speciality.*
	Can support students by directing them to learning opportunities and wider networks of learners. May facilitate seminars and workshops your student could attend. Can support learners achieving proficiencies by accessing other areas.
	Can help you to develop your skills; support you with your development; provide a different viewpoint; and/or advise on student learning matters.
Education lead/ director of education	*A senior figure within an organisation or department. The role is likely to involve: managing education provision across an organisation or area planning, delivering and evaluating a range of programmes to meet strategic and operational needs; working with a range of staff to identify future education and workforce requirements; providing advice on provision; providing advice to the organisation on improving the quality of education.*
	Supports students by strategically working to plan learning experiences across the wider organisation. Works in partnership with AEIs and supporting curriculum development.
	Can support you by providing training and development opportunities to further your skills and by providing networking opportunities for you to meet with other supervisors/assessors and lecturers from the AEI.
Link lecturer/ placement support	*Employed and based at an AEI as an academic. The role commonly involves a point of connection between the AEI and practice area to support students' practice-based learning.*
	Supports the student by being the contact for the AEI while on placement, assisting with issues and queries.
	Can support you with student issues and queries; assessment and failing matters; quality processes; your professional development; and updating you on curriculum matters.
Course leader/ programme leader/course director	*Employed and based at an AEI as an academic with the responsibility for academic leadership, management and assessment for the course they have been designated to lead.*
	Supports the student by responding to feedback from students, external examiners, Professional, Statutory and Regulatory Bodies (PSRBs) and industry.
	Can support you by providing updates and workshops and involving you in educational and curriculum development opportunities, to help your professional development.

Roles	Definition and support offered
Personal tutor/ academic advisor	*Employed and based at an AEI as an academic with the remit of providing academic and professional development support to their allocated students.* Supports students to make decisions in relation to their course, formulating plans to support their academic and personal/professional development. They connect the student with other academics and opportunities as well as with other support services as appropriate. Can support you with particular student issues by providing further information about the student as appropriate or signposting the student to other services and processes.
Academic assessor	*Employed and based at an AEI as an academic with the NMC remit of reviewing the student's performance with regards to their achievement of proficiencies and programme learning outcomes prior to progression.* Will not have a role in supervising the student in practice, teaching, assessing theoretical work or as an academic advisor for the student for the part of the programme being assessed. However, they will meet with the student at course progression points. Can communicate with practice assessors about assessment decisions relating to progression.
Student support services/student support officers/ pastoral support	*Employed and based at an HEI to provide confidential, impartial help and support to students, prospective students and graduates.* Supports the student by signposting to specialised support services including: student help; student funding; international student; careers and employability; disabled student access; wellbeing and multi-faith services. Can also support the student with AEI processes, for example absence monitoring and assessment submission. Can support you by directing your student to specialised services.
Students' Union	*Organisation which promotes, defends and extends the rights of students.* Supports the student by offering a professional, impartial, confidential and non-judgemental service, providing advice, support and representation to help resolve problems. Also provides networking opportunities, access to societies and clubs, friendship groups and extra-curricular opportunities that can develop employability skills. Can support you by directing your student to specialised services.

Table 1.2 Roles involved in supporting the student in the clinical area

The link lecturer role has long been associated with supporting student nurses and midwives in clinical practice. It is worth further consideration as it is critically placed to bridge the gap between clinical practice and AEIs. There has been a long-standing academic discussion about the link lecturer role, as there is little consistency regarding its purpose, objective and contribution to practice-based learning (MacIntosh, 2015).

The new SSSA (NMC, 2018b) have removed the requirement of the registrant teacher qualification and thus the future of the link lecturer role is increasingly unclear. For AEIs who choose to keep this type of role and use registrant lecturers in a more strategic remit, the role has the potential to flourish. In particular, the value of this role could be in helping consistent and timely communications by being the 'face' of the AEI for busy practitioners in practice. They can also support the preparation and continued professional development of supervisors and assessors and provide a valuable link to the students' curricula. Even where this role doesn't exist, there will still be partnership working opportunities as AEIs and practice learning partners are required to work collaboratively with students and service users throughout any NMC programme of study.

Students benefit from this wider network of support as they can learn from multiple perspectives and combine ideas. Practice supervisors and/or assessors also benefit from opportunities to connect and learn from others. Sylvie, introduced in this chapter, makes use of the wider network to help her to develop different perspectives on the workbook content (Activity 1.3); this will add to her resources, as she gets a range of insights and perspectives. Supporting students as a team embeds a collaborative culture required for the shared goal of student progression.

Models of organising student support in practice areas

There is a shortage in supply of qualified nurses and midwives in the UK and this has an effect on ambitious plans to deliver healthcare. As well as the NMC revising the way student nurses and midwives should be supported in clinical practice, there are other drivers for developing new models of student support such as increasing the numbers of students wanting to become health and social care professionals. The *NHS Long Term Plan* was published in 2019 by NHS England and sets out ways that care will be improved over a ten-year period. The Plan recognises that to achieve these ambitions there will be challenges to overcome, including staffing shortages. This will be addressed by 'Backing Our Workforce', which involves continuing to increase the NHS workforce, training and recruitment of more professionals. It is acknowledged this will mean thousands more clinical placements needed for undergraduate nurses.

Increasing the NHS workforce also involves reducing attrition, or student dropout, from pre-registration programmes. Of equal importance is ensuring that the students who graduate are resilient and recruited and retained in the workforce. Organisations and education providers have begun to work together differently to attract and retain the right students and to ensure they provide a high-quality clinical learning environment. This is also reflected in *Raising the Bar. Shape of Caring: A Review of the Future Education and Training of Registered Nurses and Care Assistants* (Willis and Shape of Caring Review, 2015).

However, since the start of the COVID-19 pandemic, the NHS has experienced significant and high-profile public support and there has been an unprecedented interest in NHS careers. The number of visitors to a webpage on the NHS 'Health Careers' website, which includes information on how to start a career as a nurse in the NHS, rose by 138 per cent between March and June 2020. This led to a substantial rise in students enrolling onto healthcare courses in September 2020. In August 2020 Health Education England committed funding to provide an additional 7,000 nursing and midwifery placements across all regions. This has led to a number of projects, supported by Health Education England, where organisations are trialling ways to increase placement capacity.

A large-scale project in the East of England set out to improve the quality and increase capacity within practice learning environments. Relevant publications relating to placement support and clinical learning were reviewed and from this several new approaches were developed and piloted. One of these is the Collaborative Learning in Practice (CLiP) model. Perhaps you work in an area where this has been adopted or piloted?

CLiP is based on the coaching approach, where the focus is on developing students' confidence, competence and performance through practice support. Students are expected to take responsibility for their learning while their coach encourages them to identify their own learning needs and requirements. The coach has responsibility for the quality of the learning experience (Lobo et al., 2014). This model supports the SSSA (NMC, 2018b) as the 'coach' and 'practice supervisor' are a similar role. A practice assessor steps in at the relevant assessment points, but the supervisor is responsible for the day-to-day learning.

From the evaluations of the models available to date (Clarke et al., 2018), it seems that there are six common principles in these emerging approaches to organising student support in practice areas:

1. A coaching approach is useful.
2. Support should be provided by a team – responsibility for practice learning and assessment decisions should not be with one individual.
3. Students should be delivering hands-on care – supervisors supporting the student to provide care is at the heart of new approaches.
4. Strong leadership is required for sustained change.
5. New approaches require a sustainable infrastructure.
6. Linking pre-registration education and workforce supply directly into an organisation's business agenda is helpful to maintain the profile.

CLiP has been adopted in many areas, and it is important to note that other models of organising placement learning also exist. Perhaps you have been involved in your practice setting with trying out new ways of organising student support? As well as innovations in practice supervision models, other innovations being trialled include using simulation-based learning opportunities; using technology to develop remote placement experiences; streamlining how placements are allocated; and opening up new placement opportunities. If you are interested in finding out more about Health Education England's placement expansion work, there is a link in the further reading at the end of this chapter. Activity 1.4 provides an opportunity for you to identify student support mechanisms in your own clinical practice area.

Activity 1.4   Leadership and management reflection

Each organisation will have its own unique approach to organising student support. As a practice supervisor and/or assessor, it is critical you recognise mechanisms for organising student support in your area.

1. Look at Figure 1.1. Consider the student support network for your own practice area. It will be helpful for you to make a note of this for your future reference.
2. Consider which (if any) models of organising student support exist or might be useful in your practice area.*

* You may need to speak to experienced colleagues in your practice area to help you with this activity.

There is no model answer for this activity as it relates to your own experience.

It is clear there is a need to explore different ways of supporting students to ensure they have high-quality learning experiences without compromising patient safety and patient care. In Activity 1.4 you will have identified approaches to organising student support in your own practice setting. CLiP and many other models of supporting students seem to have a common element of having a coaching approach. A coaching approach fits well with the SSSA (NMC, 2018b). Coaching is well established in the sporting world, and describes a relationship where someone trains others through instructing them and giving them advice. In relation to practice-based education, the term describes an interactive and facilitative process where a student is supported to acquire and develop skills and abilities needed for their profession by an experienced registrant over a given time period (Kelton, 2014). If you are interested in exploring coaching methods and how these could enhance your practice supervisor and/or assessor role, check out the book by Cox et al. (2014). Details are provided in the further reading section of this chapter. Also, coaching approaches are explored further in Chapter 6 of this book.

Chapter summary

This chapter has introduced the roles and responsibilities of the practice supervisor and practice assessor. These roles emerged from the NMC SSSA (NMC, 2018b) which replaced the SLAiP (NMC, 2008). These standards bring with them many changes that will be explored further in this book. Sylvie and Aleksandra and the chapter activities have attempted to bring these NMC standards to life by applying them to a range of situations. The chapter considered how reflective practice and reflective models might enhance your skills as a supervisor and/or assessor. In particular, we looked at how Sylvie had used Gibbs' model (1988) to guide her reflective practice and structure her reflective account for her NMC revalidation (2017a). The wider team supporting student practice learning was identified, including the roles you are likely to encounter. The chapter concluded with consideration of new and emerging models of organising student support in practice areas.

Activity answers

Activity 1.1: Critical thinking (p6)

1. It is not clear whether Aleksandra has been suitably prepared to take on the role of practice supervisor. She would need preparation for the role, which is the responsibility of her employing organisation. It is likely that Sylvie will support her preparation for the role, as she is an experienced mentor and preceptor. She would need to work with Sylvie and other colleagues to identify opportunities to both reflect on and develop her role as supervisor. Furthermore, she would need to be familiar with the proficiencies and programme outcomes for the students she supervises.

2. If she meets the criteria outlined above, she can supervise the full range of pre-registration students.

3. Aleksandra cannot make decisions about a student's achievement of proficiencies as this is the role of the practice assessor. However, her feedback on the student's competence should be taken into account by the assessor to make judgements about achievement and progression.

Activity 1.2: Critical thinking (p10)

1 and 2.   Yes, it is likely from the Scenario that Sylvie could be a practice supervisor and a practice assessor. However, in accordance with the SSSA, she cannot act as a supervisor to those students she is allocated to assess.

3.   As we know that Sylvie has previously completed an NMC-approved mentor course, and is already an experienced mentor, this will have prepared her to act in either of the roles. However, she will need to have access to ongoing support and training for the roles; demonstrate her continuing professional development; and be familiar with programme proficiencies and outcomes for the students she is assessing.

Activity 1.3: Critical thinking (p11)

1. You may have noted some or all of these activities for Sylvie's action plan.

    *   Evaluate the workbook – The final workbook is completed and has been signed off for use by the Trust's management team. Sylvie has offered to evaluate the workbook over the next six months.

- Staff development – As part of the developing team, we can assume Sylvie would be involved in working with colleagues on how to use the workbook.

- Disseminate the findings – As part of the developing team, we can assume Sylvie would talk to colleagues in her organisation about the new workbook and how it has been developed. As part of her role in the evaluation, she would be required to **disseminate** the findings of the evaluation through a report, and potentially through presentations or publications.

- Networking – Sylvie will need to carry on working with others as part of the evaluation and to be able to continually develop the workbook.

2. You may have noted some or all of these standards from Sylvie's reflection.

- 6 – Always practise in line with the best available evidence.

- 7 – Communicate clearly.

- 8 – Work cooperatively.

- 9 – Share your skills, knowledge and experience for the benefit of people receiving care and your colleagues.

- 20 – Uphold the reputation of your profession at all times.

- 22 – Fulfil all registration requirements.

Further reading

Howatson-Jones, L (2016) *Reflective Practice in Nursing.* London: Sage/Learning Matters.

This book supports the reader in discovering how you can apply principles of reflection to enhance your practice, patient care and professional development.

Cox, E, Bachkirova, T and Clutterbuck, DA (eds) (2014) *The Complete Handbook of Coaching.* London: Sage.

This book provides a useful guide to coaching that can be applied to a range of different professions and settings. It is aimed at helping new coaches develop their own personal style of coaching, building on approaches explained from coaching theory.

Useful websites

Supporting information on the *Standards for Student Supervision and Assessment* (SISSSA) (NMC, 2018b): **www.nmc.org.uk/supporting-information-on-standards-for-student-supervision-and-assessment**.

These pages contain supporting information from the NMC in relation to the new standards regarding student supervision and assessment and it is updated regularly.

Health Education England placement expansion and innovation resources: **www.hee.nhs.uk/our-work/allied-health-professions/helping-ensure-essential-supply-ahps/placement-expansion-innovation/resources**.

These pages contain examples of resources from projects relating to placement expansion and innovation. There are examples, frameworks, policies and presentations shared through these pages, which are updated as new projects unfold.

Learning culture

Standards Framework for Nursing and Midwifery Education (NMC, 2018d)

This chapter will address the standard: **1: Learning culture**.

1.1 the learning culture prioritises the safety of people, including carers, students and educators, and enables the values of the Code (NMC, 2015) to be upheld.

1.2 education and training is valued in all learning environments.

The Code: Professional Standards of Practice and Behaviour for Nurses and Midwives (NMC, 2015)

This chapter most closely aligns with the following professional standards.

Prioritise people

2.1 work in partnership with people to make sure you deliver care effectively.

Practise effectively

8.1 respect the skills, expertise and contributions of your colleagues, referring matters to them when appropriate.

9.1 provide honest, accurate and constructive feedback to colleagues.

9.4 support students' and colleagues' learning to help them develop their professional competence and confidence.

11.1 only delegate tasks and duties that are within the other person's scope of competence, making sure that they fully understand your instructions.

11.2 make sure that everyone you delegate tasks to is adequately supervised and supported so they can provide safe and compassionate care.

(Continued)

(Continued)

Preserve safety

15.3 take account of your own safety, the safety of others and the availability of other options for providing care.

16 act without delay if you believe that there is a risk to patient safety or public protection (16.1–16.6).

19.1 take measures to reduce as far as possible the likelihood of mistakes, near misses, harm and the effect of harm if it takes place.

19.4 take all reasonable personal precautions necessary to avoid any potential health risks to colleagues, people receiving care and the public.

Promote professionalism and trust

20 uphold the reputation of your profession at all times (20.1–20.10).

23.1 cooperate with any audits of training records, registration records or other relevant audits that we may want to carry out to make sure you are still fit to practise.

25.2 support any staff you may be responsible for to follow the Code at all times. They must have the knowledge, skills and competence for safe practice; and understand how to raise any concerns linked to any circumstances where the Code has been, or could be, broken.

Chapter aims

After reading this chapter, you will be able to:

- understand how to create and maintain a learning culture which prioritises the safety of patients and students, service users and carers;
- be able to describe what makes a good learning environment and placement learning experience;
- be able to support a diverse range of students in your practice area;
- be able to identify the role yourself and others play in creating opportunities for interprofessional collaboration.

The NMC will only approve and support programmes where the learning culture is ethical, open and honest, and conducive to safe and effective learning that respects the principles of equality and diversity, and where innovation, interprofessional learning and team working are embedded (NMC, 2018d). This chapter begins by looking at the increasingly diverse range of students in practice areas. We meet Jethro, an experienced practice supervisor in a community team, who is supporting several students, and explore his role in promoting a positive learning culture. We also consider students' individual needs, including those with a disability who may need additional support while on placement. We then focus on the standards that relate to governance and how to create and maintain a safe learning environment and then consider how we can increase opportunities to work collaboratively and interprofessionally. The chapter concludes by outlining how you can effectively use evidence to enhance your effectiveness as a practice supervisor and/or practice assessor.

The diversification of students

Diversification can apply to the *types* of students we work with as well as the unique requirements, preferences and characteristics of our students. Registered nurses and midwives have a history of supporting a wide range of students in practice including student nurses, student midwives, overseas nurses and ex-registrants who are wishing to 'return to practice'. However, greater diversification of the healthcare workforce is underway, both within and outside the nursing profession. You may already be working with new types of healthcare workers such as nursing associates, nurse apprentices, advanced clinical practitioners and physician associates, and over the next years you will see the arrival of a wider range of colleagues. In addition, you might find yourself working with students from schools and colleges or volunteering schemes.

Apprenticeships for registrant roles are becoming a popular route into healthcare as they require the student to have less time away from the workplace as they follow a work-based learning (WBL) approach. There are many definitions of WBL, but the following sums it up: learning for work, learning at work, learning from work (Burton and Jackson, 2003). WBL builds on **experiential learning** theory, which is described in Chapter 4. Apprentices will spend most of their time in the workplace, with a requirement for at least 20 per cent of their time to be engaged in 'off-the-job training', which describes the theoretical component. This is a different approach to the standard degree routes for nurse and midwifery education. Many apprentices may be established employees, possibly nursing assistants etc., so while they may be familiar with the clinical area and colleagues, they will need to adapt to a new role and acquire skills and knowledge to meet proficiencies. Practice supervisors need to support apprentices to transition into this type of student role and ensure that their time for learning is not eroded with work responsibilities (Rosser, 2017). The ability to facilitate learning on the job and apply practice experience to theory is essential when supporting this type of student.

As well as diversification in the *types* of learners, there is also increasing diversification in learner needs and expectations. For example, nursing students receive their tuition funding and financial support through the standard student support system, accessing student loans. This change in funding, from commissioned student to self-funder, may have an impact on how they perceive their role as a student nurse and their expectations of both their placement experience and the support they receive from their supervisors and assessors. This experience might be very different from when we were students. For example, students might be reluctant to work weekends or nights as they have other part-time work or caring commitments. Therefore, you will need to be adaptable and demonstrate resilience to successfully support the range of students you will encounter. Activity 2.1 offers you the opportunity to look at the students in your practice area.

Activity 2.1   Critical thinking

Who's who in your clinical area?

Take a look around your practice area; you may be working on a ward, outpatient clinic, a community setting or in primary care. Notice how many and what types of students access your practice area. Make a list and identify if they are already registrants (e.g. advanced clinical practitioners); their disciplines; where they are in their student journey; and whether they are preparing to become one of the new types of healthcare workers such as physician associates. Are they studying for a traditional degree or an apprenticeship, how are they studying (i.e. part-time, full-time, distance learning, apprenticeship routes) and what courses?

Now think about your colleagues and consider their role and responsibilities with regards to supporting students. Are they, for example, in an 'enhanced role' such as a practice educator or lecturer practitioner, or are they practice assessors or practice supervisors? Now identify any unique and shared features and how you can complement this skillset in your role as a supervisor and/or assessor.

There is no model answer to this activity as it is based on your own experiences.

Developing a diverse workforce within the NHS is hugely important. Over 22 per cent of the 1.3 million people who work in the health service are from a Black, Asian and Minority Ethnic (BAME) background, and without them the NHS wouldn't be able to function (**www.ethnicity-facts-figures.service.gov.uk/workforce-and-business/ workforce-diversity/nhs-workforce/latest**). But diversity is much wider than an individual's ethnic background and involves many other protected characteristics. Let us further consider what we mean by supporting diversity of *individuals* in our learning environments. Equality, Diversity and Inclusion (EDI) are terms often used together in the workplace and this abbreviation is used in this book. The Equality and Human Rights Commission describes equality as ensuring every individual has an equal opportunity to make the most of their lives and talents. It is also the belief that no one should have poorer life chances because of where they were born, where they came from, what they believe, who they choose to love or whether they have a disability. NHS England describes diversity as recognising and valuing differences through inclusion, regardless of age; disability; gender; racial origin; religion; belief; sexual orientation; commitments outside of work; part-time or shift work; language; union activity; HIV status; perspectives; opinions, and values.

Inclusion is taking an approach to our work where we consider individuals, their diversity, their preferences and their abilities. Health Education England defines EDI in relation to the workplace as: creating an environment where everyone can be themselves and feel that they can contribute their views, which will be valued. This is mandated by legislation including *The Health and Social Care Act* (2012), *The Equality Act* (2010) and protecting employees from employer harassment: *The Equality Employment Regulations* (2006). EDI is at the core of health- and social care-related policies and guidance. The organisation you work for will have EDI strategies or frameworks, and you should be able to easily access these. To find out more about EDI, follow the link to the Health Education England 'Diversity and Inclusion' resource at the end of this chapter.

Promoting these values in health and social care is hugely important, as everyone should be able to access the relevant services they require. A workforce should be as diverse as the population it serves, to be able to provide quality care. When we apply this principle to a learning culture, every student should have equal access to support and opportunities and learning should not be restricted by an individual's characteristics.

Your critical thinking in Activity 2.1 might have resulted in you more clearly recognising the many different students in your area, each with a range of needs, strengths, expectations and concerns. Also, you will have identified your colleagues who have a part to play in supporting them, and there will be some overlap in their roles. Practice learning environments need to offer students the best experiences possible while protecting the patient and the student. A large part of your role as practice supervisor/practice assessor is about making this happen. Scenario 2.1 outlines the diverse range of students that practice supervisors and practice assessors support.

Scenario 2.1

Central 1 comprises a large, integrated community team in the city. There is a significant number of staff working in Central 1 and a wide range of students who have varying lengths of placements. Central 1 links closely with the medical and mental health wards from the nearby hospital and students from these areas often visit for short periods of time in order to gain experience of community and integrated working. Jethro is a registered nurse and an experienced practice supervisor. He is responsible for ensuring Central 1 is an effective learning environment for all

(Continued)

(Continued)

students. He has worked there for several years and has a good working relationship with the two universities at which the majority of students are studying. Recently, he has noticed that the student population is more diverse, both in demographic make-up and the courses they are studying. His colleagues are feeling a little confused by the wide range of courses the students are undertaking and, at times, unclear as to how best to support them. Earlier in the week, he overheard one of his senior colleagues speaking on the phone, explaining that Central 1 was an unsuitable environment for a student with a hearing impairment. He also is aware that another nurse in his team has told students that they cannot swap shifts that have been allocated.

Scenario 2.1 is typical of many busy clinical areas and can place increased pressure on staff to effectively support students, including those with a disability.

'**Reasonable adjustments**' duty was first introduced under the Disability Discrimination Act in 1995. This describes an employer's responsibility to avoid, as far as possible by reasonable means, the disadvantage a disabled employee experiences because of their disability. For students, Approved Educational Institutions (AEIs), in partnership with practice learning partners, should take positive steps to ensure that disabled students can fully participate in the education and other benefits, facilities and services provided for students.

Literature studies suggest that students sometimes feel securing reasonable adjustments on placements can be difficult because of confusion over the process and whose responsibility it is. Although there is little guidance about how to best support student nurses with a disability during placement, the general consensus is that these students are more likely to succeed if they disclose early on what requirements or adjustments they need (Tee et al., 2010). Although some students may be reluctant to do this, it is important that the benefits are outlined to them and support offered should they experience problems receiving any adjustments or support on placement. Students are not obliged to disclose disabilities or impairments, unless they could cause risk, but are encouraged to do so from the time of application, to obtain assistance during the course. In Scenario 2.1, Jethro is rightly concerned that a senior colleague was overheard speaking with the AEI stating Central 1 is an unsuitable environment for a student with a hearing impairment. Jethro is sure that a student with a hearing impairment could be supported in Central 1. Good practice would be to discuss any requirements needed at a pre-placement meeting with the student's academic assessor or personal tutor to provide an opportunity for any adjustments to be put in place. At the start of the placement, these would be included in any personal learning plan, with input from both the practice area and the AEI. AEIs will have a designated person or team who specialise in supporting students with disabilities and have expertise around potential adjustments.

The Royal College of Nursing (RCN) in their publication 'Reasonable adjustments: the peer support service guide for members affected by disability in the workplace' (2017) suggest the following are common types of reasonable adjustments:

- Equipment – such as voice-activated software or an ergonomic mouse.
- Changes to working patterns – such as shift patterns, working from home and working nearer home.
- Changes to the workplace environment – such as automatic doors or altered lighting.
- Training – to educate colleagues and change attitudes.
- Re-deployment – which means moving to another more suited role that becomes available when you can't continue in your current role.
- Disability-related sickness targets (in addition to general sickness targets) – so that individuals can have time off for regular needs related to a disability.

In 2020, NHS Employers published a guide called 'How to embed flexible working for nurses'. Their research found that offering flexible working is one of the ways to attract and retain a diverse workforce, across a range of settings. It outlines common misconceptions and confirms that increasing opportunities to work flexibly hold great potential to improve nursing turnover rates and reduce the number of nurse vacancies in the NHS. The research to inform this guide found that common reasons for wanting to work flexibly included:

- improved work–life balance
- to fulfil caring responsibilities
- to suit extra-curricular activities
- to study or complete qualifications
- health reasons.

These same reasons will apply to students also, and research suggests that many student nurses and midwives have part-time jobs to support their studies or have significant caring commitments. Of course, this does not mean that students could opt to be in practice for certain times, but as practice supervisor/practice assessor you might be aware of flexible working requirements for your student. Maintaining an open dialogue can allow students to have better input in their working patterns, and encourages shared decision-making, which tends to increase commitment and attainment. Compromises can be achieved to balance the student's requests against those of the learning environment, taking into account the learning outcomes.

In Scenario 2.1, Jethro's colleague could explore with the AEI if any equipment might be useful for the student with a hearing impairment, to enable them to experience Central 1. Examples could be equipment so they could use a stethoscope, or an amplified telephone. With regards to adjustments in working patterns, the student may be allocated a particular geographical area served by Central 1, so that they become as familiar as possible with the environment. This colleague could be supported to explore flexible working patterns with her students, understanding the individual's reasons for the request and the requirements of Central 1. As part of Jethro's responsibilities for ensuring Central 1 is an effective learning environment for all students, he can ensure he provides the team with information and resources about the courses the students are undertaking and their learning requirements. The following sections in this chapter will help you to identify effective strategies for creating and maintaining an effective learning environment, while valuing learning and creating opportunities for collaboration.

Creating and maintaining a safe learning environment

This section focuses on how you, as a practice supervisor/practice assessor, can create and maintain a safe and effective learning environment for students. A well-planned induction can have a huge impact on student experience. Factors such as receiving timely information prior to the start of placement, being welcomed by the team and having 'bite-size', clear activities and objectives are very important to students during the first couple of weeks on a placement. In Activity 2.2 we look at how Jethro from the earlier Scenario can support a range of students, including those who are at the beginning of their placement.

Activity 2.2   Critical thinking

Saskia is a second-year student specialist community public health nurse (SCPHN). She is confident and highly motivated. This is her first week on Central 1. Devlin is a third-year student nurse. He has had a community placement before and is familiar with the environment; he thinks it is the area he wishes to work in when he qualifies. He has been on Central 1 for five weeks. . Rhian is a first-year Trainee Nurse Associate (TNA). She is on her first ever placement, although she worked as a healthcare support worker for ten years on a medical ward. She appears very confident and tells Jethro she can be left unsupervised, even though she has never worked in the community setting.

How can Jethro create and maintain an environment that meets the needs of this diverse range of students? What are the 'essentials' he needs to put in place for this to happen? You may wish to list five to ten 'essentials' for Jethro to implement on Central 1.

There is a model answer at the end of this chapter.

As highlighted in Activity 2.2, the clinical placement must be adaptable in order to meet students' needs. Learners will be at varying levels of experience and expertise and will have a range of proficiencies to meet. The placement should offer learning opportunities for all, and one way of achieving this is to create peer-to-peer learning opportunities.

This is where students work together on a problem or scenario to resolve issues and create solutions; for example, a supervisor may be supporting a number of students during a busy shift. The practice supervisor can present scenarios and assign specific roles and responsibilities both to individual students and to them as a team. In this way they are able to meet their individual proficiencies and learn from each other through practising team-working and communication skills. Let us consider this further in Scenario 2.2.

Scenario 2.2

It is Friday afternoon and a young mum presents at Central 1 complaining of feeling lethargic and with a rash to her face and neck. She is accompanied by her two children aged 4 years and 12 months, respectively. The children's cheeks are also red and the younger one appears drowsy. The practice supervisor, Jethro, decides to involve the students in the care of this family. He spends time with them as a group asking what they think needs to be done and to prioritise any interventions. He asks them to make a note about their decisions and the rationale for their choices. He then gets them to share this with each other and then to agree, as a group, how to care for the family. Jethro reviews their plan and makes any necessary amendments, informing the group what he has done and why. He points them to a couple of resources they can access to deepen their knowledge in these areas. Next, they agree who will undertake which activities and he arranges for them to feed back later in the day. As part of this they will provide feedback to each other about their performance and what they learnt, advising them to use a reflective model. Jethro is aware that there is a range of competence and experience in the group and also how much supervision each requires, and he makes sure that he or a colleague is available to support them.

This Scenario highlights the fact that students are a fantastic resource as they can support each other and develop their competence through team working. Involving students in peer-to-peer learning more closely replicates the 'real' world, where much care is delivered in a team environment. It is also an effective and efficient way to support a diverse range of students. Learners report that they learn significant amounts from their peers when in placement. This type of learning is often referred to as problem-based learning and it has been found to be a highly effective strategy in nurse education, especially when applied to the clinical context (Wosinski et al., 2018).

Learning culture and patient safety

Ensuring that a learning environment promotes patient safety is essential to a good learning experience. In this section we will look at three areas of patient safety: human factors, consent and duty of candour. We begin with human factors.

Human factors is an area of patient safety that has been applied to healthcare, including nurse education, from a diverse range of areas such as engineering and aviation. Human factors are things that affect an individual's performance and, as a result, have an impact on patient safety. The area focuses on the micro and macro factors including person-to-person interactions, decision-making and creating safe environments in which to work with the aim of improving practice to avoid mistakes and near misses (Fawcett and Rhynas, 2014). Organisations and placement areas that promote human factors give 'permission' to be open about near misses and mistakes, thereby promoting a learning culture that is essential to patient safety (RCN, n.d.). Human factors are seen as essential to healthcare to such an extent that the NMC has embedded human factors into the standards of proficiency for registered nurses: now all students wishing to register with the NMC must achieve this proficiency. The NMC defines human factors as "the environmental organisational and job factors, and human and individual characteristics, which influence behaviour at work in a way which can affect health and safety" (NMC, 2018a, p39). It is well recognised that patient safety is 'everybody's business' as decisions are rarely made in a **uni-professional** vacuum. Therefore, to really improve patient safety, and understand the complex human factors that are at play in the healthcare environment, education and training needs to be coordinated and delivered interprofessionally (RCN, n.d.).

A human-factors approach to patient safety starts with an understanding of the things that support or hinder the way we work. Students who are new to a practice environment can be a fantastic resource as they will notice things that others who have worked there for some time may not. In many ways they can be a 'barometer of patient safety'. As a supervisor/assessor you can improve patient safety by actively seeking their feedback and looking for ways to improve. Also, students should be involved in any learning that takes place as a result of near misses and mistakes. Often students are excluded from post-incident debriefs and learning, but including them will not only enhance their own learning (and therefore protect future patients) but also enhance the culture and practice of the clinical area.

Students, no matter where they are in their learning journey, will be familiar with the importance of reflecting on practice. In your role as supervisor/assessor you can support them to develop this to enhance patient safety. A study undertaken in Sweden found that using a three-step model of reflection, following simulated learning, demonstrated enhanced learning and attitudes (Lestander et al., 2016). The model included written and verbal reflections: steps 1 and 3 are written reflections and step 2 is a verbal group reflection. The findings demonstrated an increased commitment to patient safety and showed the value of making a mistake in the simulated scenario as the learning would help the students prepare for future situations. The pre-registration standards (NMC, 2018a, 2018e, 2019b) place a greater emphasis on the value of simulation in student learning. Simulation is a valuable and authentic learning mode which can occur in AEIs or practice areas. Activity 2.3 considers the opportunities for simulation in your area.

Activity 2.3 Decision-making

Review your student's practice assessment documents and their learning goals for the placement.

1. Make a list of the proficiencies that might best be met by simulated learning activities (this may be because there is little or no opportunity to practise them in 'real life' or the learning may be enhanced through simulation, for example creating a patient safety scenario for the students to work on together).
2. Identify which proficiencies might be best achieved via simulated learning. You may wish to view the evidence base for this and look for policies and practice in your workplace. Identify one or two from this list. (We suggest you start with something that might be easy to accomplish and not requiring too much resource: a win–win).
3. Now think about how you will deliver this learning activity. Ask yourself: Where? When? How? Who? What resources are required? Are there any obstacles?
4. Deliver the activity.*
5. Reflect on what went well and what could be done differently and share this learning with colleagues.

*There may be a nurse academic, for example a link lecturer, at the AEI who could support you to deliver the activity and work on any enhancements.

There is no model answer for this activity as this is based on your own experiences.

Activity 2.3 looked at simulation as an educational strategy to improve patient safety. This next section looks at informed consent, which is an important aspect of patient safety and maintaining a safe learning environment for patients and students.

Central to managing risk is information-giving and consent-seeking. Practice supervisors need to demonstrate to their students how to convey often complex information, check understanding and gain consent. These are complex yet subtle skills and the supervisors must make these overt to enable the student to acquire them. Prior to an interaction with a patient, you should talk through with your students the information you are sharing, how you intend to share it and how you will check understanding and gain consent. Make it clear what the goals of the interaction are and how they relate to the patient's care plan. Unfortunately, some students report that the practice of consent-seeking can be highly variable. This can lead to missed opportunities for engaging in patient care, especially in relation to an intimate or invasive procedure (Carson-Stevens et al., 2013). Chapter 3 discusses consent in relation to students being involved in an individual's care, so you may wish to review this now.

Another key factor in patient safety is 'duty of candour', and this goes hand in hand with information-giving and consent-seeking. The duty of candour of healthcare professionals and organisations was introduced in 2015 following the recommendation of the 2013 Francis Inquiry (NHS Executive, 2015). It means that as nurses we must be honest and discuss with patients when things have gone wrong, have caused harm or have the potential to do so and inform managers of adverse incidents and 'near misses' (NMC, n.d.). The duty of candour extends to healthcare organisations too; they must support staff to report near misses and adverse events and ensure there are clear mechanisms to do so. This is because organisations that support staff to speak up when things go wrong are more able to learn from mistakes and to better protect patients from harm. All NHS Trusts will be required to publish a charter for openness and transparency so that staff have clear expectations of how they will be treated if they witness and report clinical errors (Glasper, 2016). You may wish to look at the NMC's guidance on escalating concerns (NMC, 2017c) and your organisation's information about duty of candour and share these with students.

Students need to be empowered to act if they witness behaviours and practice that are harmful. Role models are powerful in this context, and Standard 3.1 of the SSSA (NMC, 2018d) states: "practice supervisors serve as role models for safe and effective practice in line with their code of conduct". Your students will be observing how you behave and this may affect their behaviours and decision-making when faced with a similar scenario (Chapter 3 discusses escalation of concerns in more detail). A recent study found that practice-based mentors who can role-model professional attributes appear to be crucial in the development of professional attributes and behaviours in student nurses (Felstead and Springett, 2016). There is a detailed section on role modelling in Chapter 5.

A 'just culture' approach to patient safety

Complementing the duty of candour requirements is the 2018 *A Just Culture Guide*, produced by NHS England and NHS Improvement. This guide encourages managers of health and social care organisations to treat any staff involved in a patient safety incident in a consistent, constructive and fair way. 'Just culture' is a concept that highlights how mistakes are generally caused by faulty organisational culture, rather than caused directly by any person involved. This more macro-level perspective complements human factors and offers an alternative to a 'blame culture'. The guide encourages fair treatment of staff and a culture of fairness, openness and learning.

An important part of a 'just culture' is being clear about the approach that will be taken if an incident occurs, providing clarity and transparency. It also serves as a communication tool to help staff, learners and patients understand how the appropriate response to an incident can and should differ according to the circumstances in which an error was made. You will have established processes in place for escalating concerns and reporting incidents, and these processes are an NMC requirement for the learning environment. Any student involved in an incident or accident (or near miss) whilst on placement is required to report the event to the AEI as soon as possible. This guide does not replace the need for any of this or patient safety investigation as these all can be used as learning and improvement opportunities for the organisation. You could talk to your colleagues about how the just culture is supported in your practice area.

Learning organisations

Having considered the duty of candour requirements and just culture, another approach to promoting a learning culture is for the organisation to become a learning organisation. Learning organisations are not interested in avoidance of harm or maintenance of a steady state. Instead, they have a focus on safety and quality with a continuous improvement perspective. They are open to system-wide changes that bring about transformational care. Some learning organisations will go beyond the patient focus and aim for continuous improvement for all their employees as well, perhaps even incorporating wider civic responsibilities, such as improving the health of the communities which they serve.

Many health and social care organisations advertise that they are, or are aspiring to be, learning organisations. When employers are serious about their intention to become a learning organisation, there should be systems in place to get feedback about the services they provide. Once the feedback is obtained, there should be a clear process of how this feedback will be used. A learning organisation invests in the training and development of its staff with an emphasis on team learning and capability, as opposed to individual learning. This team learning needs to transcend artificial boundaries and networks, such as department and clinical specialities, and look to the whole organisation. Challenging people's assumptions about the world, including healthcare, allows greater learning to take place and promotes innovation. Underneath all of this is a shared vison – one that people can make sense of and buy into. Lastly, one vital yet often overlooked feature is the celebration of success and valuing achievements (Davies and Nutley, 2000). Activity 2.4 will help you to further think about the learning culture of a practice area in relation to patient safety.

Activity 2.4   Critical thinking

In Activity 2.2 we met the students Jethro was responsible for. One of them, Rhian, a first-year TNA with ten years of experience as a healthcare support worker on a medical ward, is on her first placement, and she said to Jethro that she could be left unsupervised. At the start of the shift, Jethro is surprised to witness Rhian placing a blood pressure monitor cuff around a

(Continued)

(Continued)

patient's arm and proceeding to take a reading, without any communications with the patient.

1. Should Jethro approach this incident with Rhian?
2. How should Jethro approach this incident with Rhian?
3. What are the main points he needs to raise?

There is a model answer at the end of this chapter.

Activity 2.4 applies some aspects of learning culture in relation to a patient safety example. We now consider features of the learning environment that promote a learning culture.

The learning environment and promoting a positive learning culture

Your area is more than a place in which to care for patients; it is also a learning environment – an active classroom, if you like. As a practice supervisor or practice assessor, you are instrumental in creating this learning space. We now consider how to ensure the learning environment has a learning culture and use evidence to help us consider the features of a good placement.

A learning environment can describe many different practice settings and has been defined by the RCN as a place where learning opportunities are available for students to undertake practice under the supervision of a range of practitioners in the team. It is the environment where students meet and develop therapeutic relationships with a range of patients, service users and their carers.

The NMC (2018b, p5) provides 11 standards outlining how to achieve an effective learning environment, which it defines as:

All students are provided with safe, effective and inclusive learning experiences. Each learning environment has the governance and resources needed to deliver education and training. Students actively participate in their own education, learning from a range of people across a variety of settings.

Effective learning experiences are those that put the student at the centre with opportunities to meet their learning outcome. The learning environment should provide a space for students to develop their own practice, without compromising public safety.

An effective learning experience is likely to take place across different learning environments; for example, following a patient's care journey through different hospital departments. This will allow students to learn and consolidate a set of skills across different settings and situations. Learning experiences should include the full spectrum of care relevant to the student's area or field of practice (NMC, 2018b).

In 2014, the organisation NHS Employers published *Excellence in Student Nursing Placements*, which explores the features of effective student placements based on student evaluations submitted to the *Student Nursing Times* awards relating to the 'excellent provision of placements' category. They found that placement learning is a vital part of a student's learning experience, and a good placement will contribute greatly to their development. They also noted that high-quality placements promote excellent nursing practice and a positive culture and can attract and retain staff with the right values to work in that area. The student feedback highlighted six areas that were features of a good placement:

- Compassion and other values are embedded in the team
- Time to care
- Excellent communication
- Competent leaders, mentors and colleagues
- Commitment to learning
- Courage to be flexible and to try something different.

Other studies have focused on the culture of practice learning environments to determine the factors that help and hinder learning (Lewin, 2007; Chuan and Barnett, 2012). A list of these factors is displayed in Table 2.1.

Factors that support learning	Factors that inhibit learning
Feeling welcomed	Students having to 'compete' for learning opportunities
Friendly staff	Being delegated menial tasks that do not challenge
Supervisors who are familiar with students' course and learning outcomes	The placement being too busy to enable students adequate opportunity to practise
Supervision from registered staff	Staff not interested in supervising students
Diverse learning experiences	Unfriendly staff
Peer support and learning from other students	Students who are not actively engaged in their learning

Table 2.1 Factors that influence student learning on placement

You will see from studying Table 2.1 that students feeling welcomed by friendly, approachable staff has a positive impact on their learning. Interestingly, staff often perceive their practice area to be friendlier compared with the students' perceptions. This could be for several reasons, including their familiarity with the clinical area, more established relationships and also increased confidence. Students report that rotating around different practice areas is stressful as they feel they have to 'fit in' to each new area. The learning we can take from this is that we may need to be very aware of how we welcome students onto our practice area and help them feel supportive.

It would seem that staff attitudes and behaviour exert a significant influence on the learning environment and how it is perceived by students. It is, of course, difficult to separate staff behaviours from other aspects of the learning environment, and it is acknowledged that there are a number of other factors that may have a negative influence on the learning environment, including:

- teaching and learning activities that place the students as passive recipients;
- a focus on factual recall, which can be intimidating and stifle problem-solving;
- vague objectives that are confusing and result in time being spent trying to navigate these rather than learning;
- placement areas that do not optimise the potential for **interprofessional learning** (the benefits of which are outlined in Chapter 3).

Table 2.1 outlines a number of practical issues that have a negative effect on learning; one of the most commonly cited is students feeling that they are competing for learning opportunities and tasks to enable them to meet proficiencies. This can be related to poor planning, where learning opportunities are ad hoc, resulting in an increased sense of competitiveness and anxiety in students. However, there are some quick fixes, and longer-term solutions that can address these:

- Involve a group of students in a discussion following an event or intervention. This is particularly useful when it would have been unfeasible for all students to be involved in the actual event. The post-event discussion and analysis can be an equally powerful learning experience.
- Ensure that you and the student are clear what their objectives are for the whole placement, and review these regularly.
- Plan learning opportunities with the student. Students can co-construct their learning opportunities with you. Identify the opportunities available and work with your team to maximise student involvement.
- Empower students to ask questions, make suggestions and give feedback.
- Make overt connections between theory and practice learning, e.g., "You have learnt about risk factors in relation to falls; we are now going to assess patient X to determine their risk. What are the key areas we should cover and which assessment tools should we consider using?"
- Engage all staff in student learning, including managers and senior staff. Try to create a structured learning programme into which staff from a range of professions provide input.

Toxic learning cultures

In contrast to the positive learning culture is a 'toxic' learning culture. This describes an environment where students and staff find it difficult to learn or progress because of a negative atmosphere or working conditions. Some signs that an environment is toxic are: colleagues with little or no enthusiasm for learning and/or students; risk adversity and a constant fear of making mistakes; little clarity on roles or responsibilities; ineffective communication; lack of trust amongst staff; malicious gossip; and high turnover of staff. If you recognise any of these signs, the first step in moving away from this sort of culture is to get help. If you are working in this sort of environment, it's unlikely that everyone will want to immediately support a change; however, some colleagues will, so finding allies is essential to garner support for change. If you are in a position to lead a change in culture, no matter how seemingly small, start by focusing on an aspect you can control. Rather than trying to 'fix' everything at once, plan out steps to achieve one clear change and stay focused on that aspect. For example, if you recognise that your colleagues are not clear about the SSSA roles and responsibility and this is causing confusion, set this as a focus. Get support from any interested colleagues and educate the wider team on the roles and responsibilities, perhaps working with any education leads for your organisation or enlisting the help of colleagues from other areas where this is going well. When decisions are made and plans are developed, document these so there is absolute transparency to the wider team. Providing regular feedback on progress will help keep you focused and on track. Tackling one negative aspect of a learning culture at a time will achieve change, but do expect the first steps to take time. However, once a change begins to be noticeable in the environment, this becomes positively contagious and other, often unintentional, improvements start to occur.

Activity 2.5 provides an opportunity for you to look at the strengths and limitations of your own practice area, as a learning environment.

Activity 2.5   Leadership and management

Using the information in this chapter, complete a SWOT (Strengths, Weaknesses, Opportunities, Threats) analysis of your practice learning environment. Once you have completed it, identify two short-term actions you wish to adopt.

Strengths (often internal to your organisation)	Weaknesses (often internal to your organisation)
These may be cultural such as attitudes and motivations of your colleagues	*These may be related to resources or levels of expertise and experience*

(Continued)

(Continued)

Opportunities (often external to your organisation)	Threats (often external to your organisation)
These may include the strength of the relationships with the AEI	*These could include changes or requirements imposed by external bodies or organisations*

There is no model answer for this activity as it is based on your own practice area; however, you could discuss your SWOT and two actions with colleagues in your practice setting. These could be developed into objectives for you to discuss at your appraisal and further develop.

Interprofessional collaboration

We started this chapter by asking you to consider your colleagues' role and responsibilities with regards to supporting students (Activity 2.1). You will have noted that there are usually many other people within a learning environment, no matter what the clinical setting is. Most of us will regularly work interprofessionally, alongside colleagues from different professional groups, patients, service users and carers. Throughout the chapter exploration of learning culture, it is evident that one person alone cannot create a learning culture; instead we rely on a range of people and organisational leadership to develop this. It is therefore no surprise that the learning culture requires collaborative working.

Wherever possible, interprofessional learning and working should be promoted to ensure the learning culture encompasses everyone. Interprofessional collaboration, whether it is for learning or working, occurs when two or more professions work together to achieve common goals. It is often used as a means for solving complex issues, as it improves communication, which in turn improves patient outcomes. The evidence for interprofessional collaboration overwhelmingly shows that this approach creates teams that work better together because they have a better understanding of each other's roles, increased respect and trust for each other and better task prioritisation. All these are important features in quality of care and patient safety. According to the World Health Organization (WHO, 2013, n.p.):

Collaborative practice happens when multiple health workers from different professional backgrounds work together with patients, families, carers and communities to deliver the highest quality of care across settings and improve patient experience.

This type of collaborative approach in a learning environment extends beyond interprofessional collaboration. It also involves collaborating with students, patients, service users and carers. This will promote learning from others' experiences and viewpoints and develop listening and communication skills. Engaging everyone in the learning environment also ensures a more efficient use of learning resources and learning opportunities. Collaborative learning is underpinned by social learning theories which view learning as a naturally occurring social act: learning occurs through communicating, seeking to understand the world and solving problems. These features of collaborative working are also fundamental in the steps required to build and maintain a positive learning culture.

Learning theories and interprofessional learning are explored further in Chapter 4.

Chapter summary

This chapter has identified the key components of a learning culture and features of a learning environment. We have identified the practice supervisor and practice assessor roles in preserving patient safety and explored information-giving and consent. The diverse range of students and modes of study means that there is greater complexity for supervisors and assessors. We have also explored EDI requirements ensuring the learning culture is fair and transparent and fosters good relations between individuals and diverse groups. The chapter concluded with consideration of interprofessional collaboration.

Activity answers

Activity 2.2: Critical thinking (p30)

Jethro needs to make every student feel welcome and ensure that there are learning opportunities for all. Although the team may be more experienced and familiar with supporting student nurses, they need to attend to the needs of all students such as Saskia and Rhian. Jethro could do lots of things, but here are some suggestions:

- Devise a welcome pack for all students which is not profession-specific or heavily student nurse-focused.

- Create a list of all the learning opportunities including visits and specialist practitioners; identify which students they may be most relevant to.

- Invite the link academics from the universities to visit to brief the staff on all of the types of students, their programmes and any unique needs (such as endpoint assessment).

- Provide an outline from each type of student detailing the programme they are on and what they hope to get from the placement.

- Schedule an update session familiarising the staff with the proficiencies and practice assessment documentation.

- Create an opportunity for frequently asked questions (FAQs), either face to face, online or in a student file.

- Ask supervisors who have supported these types of students to talk about their experiences and offer tips.

- Create opportunities for interprofessional learning to enable students and colleagues to learn 'with, from and about each other'.

- Develop a book, a little like a hotel guests' comments book, where past students can leave comments about their experience and the opportunities, what they found useful and what they would recommend.

Activity 2.4: Critical thinking (p35)

1. Yes, Jethro must address his concerns with Rhian.

2. Jethro is aware Rhian seems confident and has relevant prior experience, likely to involve blood pressure monitoring. However, he has not yet had an opportunity to supervise this. He has now witnessed poor practice. Jethro should ask Rhian to speak with him somewhere private. He should provide constructive feedback (information specific, issue focused) on what he has witnessed, allowing Rhian the opportunity to discuss. It is important that throughout feedback he demonstrates values of kindness, compassion and professionalism whilst providing clarity on poor practice and re-educating Rhian on good practice.

3. Rhian in her actions failed to give the patient any information on what she was about to do, and then seek the patient's consent. Jethro explains how to undertake this task by providing the patient with information, check understanding and then to gain consent for the blood pressure monitoring to be undertaken.

Further reading

Health Education England (2018) *Diversity and Inclusion: Our Strategic Framework, 2018–2022.* Available online at: **www.hee.nhs.uk/our-work/diversity-inclusion/diversity-inclusion-our-strategic-framework-2018-2022**.

NHS Employers (2014) *What Makes a Good Placement?* London: NHS Employers.

This resource contains case studies from NHS Trust placement areas that were shortlisted for the *Student Nursing Times* awards. It is mapped against the 6Cs (care, compassion, courage, commitment, communication and competence) and identifies areas of good practice. Available online at: **www.nhsemployers.org/case-studies-and-resources/2014/08/what-makes-a-good-student-placement**.

Chapter 3

Educational governance and quality

Standards Framework for Nursing and Midwifery Education (NMC, 2018d)

This chapter will address the standard: **2: Educational governance and quality**.

2.1 There are effective governance systems that ensure compliance with all legal, regulatory, professional and educational requirements, differentiating where appropriate between the devolved legislatures of the UK, with clear lines of responsibility and accountability for meeting those requirements and responding when standards are not met, in all learning environments.

2.2 All learning environments optimise safety and quality, taking account of the diverse needs of, and working in partnership with, service users, students and all other stakeholders.

The Code: Professional Standards of Practice and Behaviour for Nurses and Midwives (NMC, 2015)

This chapter most closely aligns with the following professional standards.

Prioritise people

3.4 act as an advocate for the vulnerable, challenging poor practice and discriminatory attitudes and behaviour relating to their care.

Practise effectively

8.5 work with colleagues to preserve the safety of those receiving care.

8.6 share information to identify and reduce risk.

8.7 be supportive of colleagues who are encountering health or performance problems. However, this support must never compromise or be at the expense of patient or public safety.

11.2 make sure that everyone you delegate tasks to is adequately supervised and supported so they can provide safe and compassionate care.

(Continued)

(Continued)

Preserve safety

16.4 acknowledge and act on all concerns raised to you, investigating, escalating or dealing with those concerns where it is appropriate for you to do so.

16.5 not obstruct, intimidate, victimise or in any way hinder a colleague, member of staff, person you care for or member of the public who wants to raise a concern.

16.6 protect anyone you have management responsibility for from any harm, detriment, victimisation or unwarranted treatment after a concern is raised.

Promote professionalism and trust

23.1 cooperate with any audits of training records, registration records or other relevant audits that we may want to carry out to make sure you are still fit to practise.

25.2 support any staff you may be responsible for to follow the Code at all times. They must have the knowledge, skills and competence for safe practice; and understand how to raise any concerns linked to any circumstances where the Code has been, or could be, broken.

Chapter aims

After reading this chapter, you will be clear on the roles and responsibilities of Approved Educational Institutions (AEIs) and practice learning partners in ensuring educational governance and quality in relation to:

- recruitment and selection of students;
- practice learning environment and placement opportunities;
- managing fitness to practise issues;
- managing failing students.

Introduction

Educational governance and quality are about ensuring there are processes and practices in place to protect the public and students have access to safe and effective environments in which to learn. The NMC expects education providers and practice learning partners to work together to ensure they comply with all legal and regulatory requirements. This chapter starts with student recruitment and selection requirements, then moves on to preparation for placement, including students requiring reasonable adjustments. It then looks at external factors, such as policy and regulation.

We consider what practice supervisors and practice assessors need to do to ensure a safe and effective learning environment and experience for students. The chapter concludes by focusing on professional behaviour and fitness to practise.

The responsibility for ensuring educational governance and quality spans the AEI (which is usually a university) and the practice learning environment – usually the NHS and organisations providing NHS services (NMC, 2018d). Therefore, partnership working is essential to ensure this happens effectively. Practice supervisors, practice assessors and academic assessors all have a role to play and need to communicate, work closely and understand their own and each other's roles and responsibilities, knowing who to go to for support. Scenario 3.1 introduces you to Jasper, to whom we will refer throughout this chapter.

Scenario 3.1

Jasper is a first-year student nurse who has recently started his placement experience in a dementia unit. He has not yet had much support from his practice supervisor and doesn't find the learning environment welcoming or supportive. He has felt isolated as a student. However, he is an avid user of social media and has been since starting his course.

He appreciates the immediacy social media affords, and that important discussions can be aired with huge reach. Many of the lecturers at the university use social media to engage in discussions about nursing. He is a follower of many national nurse leaders and has a significant online presence.

Most of the staff on the dementia unit don't use social media, although a couple of them use it on a personal basis to keep up with family and friends. Jasper's enthusiasm since arriving on the unit has motivated some of the team to start using social media and they now follow him on Twitter.

As we can see in Scenario 3.1, many student nurses are confident in using social media and believe it has value for progressing the nursing profession. However, not all nurses are comfortable using it, and some may be suspicious of its relevance to practice and the profession.

Concerns have been highlighted relating to the effectiveness of support for students in practice settings. These concerns are evidenced in the reports from the Shape of Caring review (Willis and Shape of Caring Review, 2015) and the RCN Mentorship Project (Royal College of Nursing, 2016b). These documents have been instrumental in the development of the NMC Educational Framework (2018b, 2018d) on which this book is based.

Before we look at Activity 3.1, read the following key recommendations from the Willis Commission (2012):

Quality with Compassion: The future of nurse education – Theme 3: Learning to nurse. (Please note: the term mentor is used throughout the document as its publication preceded the NMC Educational Framework.)

1. The quality of many practice learning experiences urgently needs improvement. Learning to care in real-life settings lies at the heart of patient-centred education and learning to be a nurse.

2. The NMC standards must be fully implemented through active partnerships between NHS education and training boards at national and local levels, employers and universities, to ensure the quality of nursing education, and use and share existing tools and standards.

3. Managers, mentors, practice education facilitators and academic staff must work together to help students relate theory to practice. Close, effective collaboration between universities and practice settings should be enhanced through joint appointments.

4. Employers and universities must together identify positive practice environments in a wide range of settings. Many more placements must be made available in community settings, including general practice. The absence of funding to higher education institutions (HEIs) to support nursing students' practical learning experiences must be addressed.

5. Employers must ensure mentors have dedicated time for mentorship, while universities should play their full part in training and updating mentors. Mentors must be selected for their knowledge, skills and motivation; adequately prepared; well supported; and valued, with a recognised status.

6. Practical learning must be underpinned with relevant knowledge from clinical and social science disciplines. All students should be aware of the growing evidence base on good nursing practice. Graduate nurses, as future leaders of clinical teams, should understand how to evaluate, utilise and conduct research, and act on evidence to improve the quality of care.

Activity 3.1 Evidence-based practice and research

After reading the recommendations from the Willis Commission (2012), identify any learning points relating to your practice supervisor/practice assessor role and decide upon one activity you can complete to address this.

There is no model answer for this activity as it is based on your own research and individual learning needs. You might find it helpful to discuss your learning from this activity with colleagues.

As a result of a range of evidence and documents, including the Willis report (2012), the education and governance of nursing and midwifery education has been over-hauled. There are two standards which account for education and governance. These are: *governance and accountability* and *safety and quality assurance*. Practice supervisor and practice/academic assessor roles are at the heart of these standards. We will consider governance and accountability first.

Governance and accountability are terms concerned with ensuring processes are in place to ensure students are both suitable for practice and placed in safe learn-ing environments which offer them the opportunities and support they require to achieve proficiencies. This can be broken down into the following areas of the stu-dent's programme:

- Recruitment and selection
- Local governance processes and orientating the student to these
- Data sharing
- Failing students.

Recruitment and selection – although it is the AEI that is responsible for recruiting students to a programme, practice learning partners have an essential role in strength-ening this. Selection processes must involve practice learning partners to ensure they are robust and select the most appropriate students. AEIs and practice learning partners work closely in the recruitment and selection of students. By taking part in recruitment and selection events, you will strengthen your skillset and contribute to your continuing professional development.

Service users and carers are also required to be part of the recruitment and selec-tion process, and work collaboratively with the AEI in programme delivery. This adds to the robustness of NMC programmes. There is the requirement that applicants meet the requirements set by the NMC, namely being of good 'health and character'. This involves applicants declaring any health condition or disability, criminal convictions and cautions. Given the NMC needs to be assured that people applying to join, renew or be readmitted to the register meet its requirements for health to ensure they can practise safely and effec-tively, it is vital they are reflected in the recruitment and selection stages. It is important to stress that this does not mean the applicant must have no prior or existing health condition and/or disability, as many people with disabilities and health conditions are able to practise effectively, with or without adjustments put in place to support them. During the COVID-19 pandemic, it has been vital for students and most registrants to undertake an enhanced occupational health screening to assess individual risk. This highlights this process as itera-tive, and certainly not something which only applies to commencing a programme.

In relation to 'good character', the NMC needs to be assured that a student is capable of safe and effective practice following completion of their programme. This includes con-sideration of any criminal proceedings, findings by another regulatory body (including health and social care) and conduct which may amount to a breach of the NMC Code.

AEIs have fitness-to-practise experts who advise on any declarations and the suitability of candidates. It is important to note that these declarations are relevant not only to the recruitment stage but throughout the programme as the Code requires all students to inform their AEI should their health and good character standing change.

The NMC has published guidance on health and character (2019a) and it is helpful to familiarise yourself with this, especially if you take part in any selection and recruitment activities.

Some students may have relevant knowledge and skills from previous learning, for example transferring between AEIs or previous relevant education. These students should have the opportunity for this to be taken into account and, where possible, be used to reduce the length of study. This is usually referred to as **recognition of prior learning (RPL)** and any claims must meet the NMC and AEI standards and regulations. You might be involved in supporting learners in your practice learning environment who are working towards an RPL claim, for example those applying to start a two-year pre-registration master's programme leading to registration with the NMC. These learners may be working towards completing a portfolio of learning that is used as part of their application.

Recruitment should be 'values-based'; this means recruiting students whose values and behaviours align with the values of the NHS Constitution (NHS England, 2015), outlined in Table 3.1.

Value	Description
Working together for patients	Patients come first in everything we do. Patients, families, service users, carers, communities should be involved in care design and delivery. NHS staff and organisations speak up when things go wrong.
Respect and dignity	Every person is valued (patients, families, service users, carers or staff) – as an individual. Views and experiences, aspirations and commitments are taken seriously. Staff are honest and open about what can and cannot be done.
Commitment to quality of care	Insist on quality and getting the basics of quality of care (safety, effectiveness, patient experience) right every time. Encouraging and welcoming feedback which is acted on to improve care and services.
Compassion	Compassion is central to care provided, we respond with humanity and kindness to each person's pain, distress, anxiety or need. This is active and not reactive.
Improving lives	We strive to improve health and wellbeing and people's experiences of the NHS and other health and social care providers. Excellence and professionalism are nurtured and celebrated. Everyone has a part to play in making ourselves, patients and communities healthier.
Everyone counts	Resources are maximised for the benefit of the whole community. No one (individual or communities) is excluded, discriminated against, or left behind.

Table 3.1   NHS Constitution values

Recruitment and selection activities should assess these values, behaviours and skills so that the students who are selected hold the right aptitude to support effective team working in order to deliver excellent patient care and experience (Health Education England, 2016). There has been an increased focus on the values held by the NHS workforce, partly as a result of the Mid-Staffordshire NHS Foundation Trust Public Inquiry (Francis, 2013), which highlighted the vital role of the workforce in providing high-quality and safe healthcare. Getting involved in recruitment and selection events will familiarise you with the whole range of expectations placed on students which help shape the future workforce. Activity 3.2 will help you do this in your practice area.

Activity 3.2   Team working

Get in touch with your link lecturer (academic contact from your students' AEI) and volunteer to take part in recruitment and selection events. Your knowledge and experience will be invaluable to the process. Familiarise yourself with the values of the NHS Constitution and the NMC guidance on health and character (2019a) before the event. Reflect on how these are being assessed in candidates, and how this meets the professional standards within the Code (NMC, 2015).

These activities will also provide you with good evidence for your appraisal/personal development review and your NMC revalidation (NMC, 2017a). Once you have attended the recruitment and selection event, complete a reflective account using the NMC revalidation template (available on the NMC website, and in Chapter 1 of this book).

There is no model answer to this activity as it is based on your own actions.

We now turn our attention to students with extra needs. As highlighted through the declaration of 'health', introduced earlier in this chapter, students may start the programme with a known health condition and/or disability which may have an impact on their learning. If this is the case, the AEI should provide them with an assessment of their needs and any support or **reasonable adjustments** to enable them to be successful in their learning (NMC, 2019a). However, students may develop a health condition or disability while undertaking the programme. It is not unusual for a student to have a learning needs assessment, for example, and be identified as having dyslexia, which may have gone unnoticed until this point. These students may need a period of adjustment in coming to terms with this and should be given all the support required to help them. They may need more time to complete tasks, access to specialist equipment or have other adjustments, such as set breaks or time to attend appointments with staff such as counsellors or occupational health services (L'Ecuyer, 2019). Supporting student diversity is explored further in Chapter 2.

AEIs have specialist services and resources for students with disabilities, therefore it is likely that students may come to your practice area with a learning contract. A learning contract is an AEI's way of recording what adjustments a student needs because of their disclosed disability or condition. Once the student has agreed to the learning contract, it is shared with relevant staff supporting the student's learning. Depending on the adjustments, this might be shared with you as practice supervisor/practice assessor, and this will be done in a timely manner to allow for any additional adjustments to be put in place. Your role is to be clear on what the student's needs are, seek clarity from the AEI if needed and then facilitate this adjustment.

You can contact the link lecturer or other academic link from the student's AEI if you are unsure how to support a student with a learning contract. Students may choose not to disclose any details of their disability. The focus should be on ensuring they have any adjustments in place by working with the AEI. It is important to protect the student's privacy in relation to this, ensuring others act respectfully and confidentially.

Local governance processes – each placement area will have a range of local governance processes in place. It is important that as practice supervisor/practice assessor you orientate your students to these, paying particular attention to information governance policies and procedures. It is good practice to make available any information that is relevant to the students prior to commencing the placement, e.g. dress code and uniform policy. Students need to be familiarised with and informed about Information Technology (IT) systems and data-sharing requirements. They also need to be informed about how to escalate concerns and the procedure for any untoward incident such as injury or assault. Completing Activity 3.3 will help you improve the information available to students.

Activity 3.3   Leadership and management

In your practice learning environment, review the information in relation to local governance processes provided to students at the start of their placement. Do you have a student handbook or file? How up to date is it? Try to look at it objectively and ask yourself how helpful this information is. If you do not have a student handbook or resource, then talk to colleagues in your workplace about creating one. You may wish to contact a colleague from the education department in your organisation to ask if there are any examples of good student resources, or a template you can use. Don't forget to talk to the students in your area and ask them to feed back on the existing resources or suggest what they might find useful to include. You will recall from Chapter 2 that a learning organisation actively seeks and responds to feedback. Try to avoid creating just a collection of documents. It is useful to include a paragraph outlining why the information has been included, how they might use it and how it might help them achieve on the placement.

There is no model answer for this activity as it is based on your own actions.

Having clear and detailed information provides clarity for everyone in the learning environment as well as evidence of the support available to students, which may be reviewed during internal and external monitoring checks, such as NMC approval events and **Care Quality Commission (CQC)** inspections.

Data sharing – practice areas and education institutions are regularly reviewed and monitored via internal processes and external bodies including the **Quality Assurance Agency (QAA)**, CQC and NMC. The outcomes of these events may have implications for student learning, and it is important you are clear about any issues identified and recommendations made. The last report from the CQC or your Trust or practice area will include a list of areas of good practice and areas to improve. General Data Protection Regulation (GDPR) came into effect in May 2018. The aim of this new legislation, which replaced the Data Protection Act, is to update and strengthen data protection regulation in the European Union (EU). The UK government has confirmed that leaving the EU will not affect the UK's compliance with GDPR as it offers best practice when handling and sharing data. This is highly relevant legislation for you as clinical practitioners but also as practice supervisors and/or practice assessors (Astrup, 2018).

Escalating concerns and failing students – of course, not every student is successful in meeting the proficiencies in practice and may fail. If this isn't something you have experienced, or haven't experienced for some time, then you may wish to familiarise yourself with the process and support available to you as a practice supervisor/practice assessor. The AEI will have clear guidance about this so get in touch with your academic contact person and ask for the information. It is much easier to digest this type of information and explore implications when you are not in the midst of managing a real-life difficult situation. Most AEIs will have processes in place for managing failing students. Vinales (2015) has created a useful algorithm which can be used by practice supervisors and practice assessors to support them in making decisions about competence. This step-by-step approach clearly identifies decision points and in doing so reduces the risks of leaving it very late before any issues around student competence are escalated. Activity 3.4 further explores issues such as fitness to practise, professional behaviours and escalating concerns.

Scenario 3.2

Jasper has been using Twitter to share his experiences on the dementia unit and how much he is learning on the placement. Now, a few weeks in, he feels much more supported by his practice supervisor and the wider team. He has a healthy number of followers on Twitter and many of his posts have been reposted. Nell, a member of the dementia unit who uses social media, reads Jasper's posts and is concerned. She thinks that some of the content makes the placement area easily identifiable and potentially breaches patient confidentiality. She speaks to Precious, Jasper's practice supervisor, about her concerns. Precious is not familiar with social media and is unsure of what she can do about this.

Social media is used regularly by students and healthcare professionals and can be a fantastic vehicle to enhance learning and professional development. There is growing literature on how the different generations (baby boomers through to Generation Z) relate uniquely to social media and this can lead to differences in opinion about its usefulness and appropriateness (Jones et al., 2015). Chapter 4 examines these generational differences. Also, social media is regularly implicated in fitness to practise and disciplinary concerns for both students and registrants. Activity 3.4 provides an opportunity for you to explore these issues, and how they might be handled.

Activity 3.4 Decision-making

Consider how Precious, from Scenario 3.2, should respond to the concerns raised by Nell. Identify three actions she could take and make a note of these.

There is a model answer for this activity at the end of the chapter.

Although Activity 3.4 is focused on Precious, Jasper's practice assessor, supporting students who are causing concern is the joint responsibility of the AEI and the practice learning environment. Students must be given opportunities to succeed, and practice and education partners must work closely to help them (see Chapter 6 for guidance on action planning in such instances). However, if, after support, a student is not competent to pass, the decision must be made to fail them (Duffy, 2003; Gainsbury, 2010). The decision that a student has passed or failed is one of the most transparent acts of accountability for the practice assessor/academic assessor and if the decision is to fail a student, this can be a stressful time for all involved. If you find yourself in this situation, it may be helpful to seek support from an experienced assessor to help you through this process (see Chapter 7 for more on this).

Safety and quality assurance are concerned with protecting the public and students by ensuring safe learning environments and promoting professional behaviours. These three areas are:

- preparing and maintaining the learning environment;
- keeping up to date with the curriculum and curriculum development;
- promoting professional behaviour.

Preparing and maintaining a safe and effective learning environment – the whole team has a role to play in this and although one person may take a lead, they rely heavily on colleagues' commitment and expertise.

Features of a learning environment are covered in Chapter 2. When considering governance processes and the learning environment, an audit of the environment ensures the area complies with all relevant legal, regulatory, professional and educational requirements. Prior to students being allocated to an area, it is a requirement that there is an up-to-date placement audit. This is undertaken jointly by the practice learning partners and the AEI. It should include details about the number and types of students who can be placed there and an agreement that there are suitably prepared and supported practice supervisors and practice assessors. In addition, the practice area must be safe and offer learning opportunities to enable the student to meet the proficiencies. Students must be able to access a range of opportunities and given time and support to develop their knowledge and skills. The AEI and NMC need to be assured that the placement can achieve all of the above to be considered as a student learning environment. Once the audit has been undertaken and agreed by both parties, then students can be allocated. There is variation across the UK as to what the audit tool looks like and where the audit is recorded, but they all contain similar information and checks. They usually cover placement learning information for nursing, midwifery and nursing associate students as well as for allied health professionals and medical students.

Practice areas must be given information by the AEI about the start and end dates of student placements and where the students are in their programme of study. The education lead in your area will usually receive this information. It is then your responsibility as practice supervisor/practice assessor to prepare for the students' arrival.

Students report that it is often the little things that make a big difference to their placement experience and learning. These can be: students being informed who their practice supervisor/practice assessor is prior to commencing; being sent information about the placement; having a shift pattern for the first week or so; and having a safe place to store their belongings (Hamshire et al., 2012). Activity 3.5 will help you identify what could make a difference for the students allocated to your practice learning environment.

Activity 3.5   Team working

Take a look at the information for your practice learning environment that is given to students before they start their placement. Make a note of what you think is helpful, and of anything that could be removed or added. Does it provide information about the clinical work, shift requirements and name of the practice assessor (and/or practice supervisor); is it friendly and welcoming in tone?

Now think about how you induct a student to your practice area. Do you have a formal induction session that all colleagues use, or is it ad hoc? Do students know their responsibilities with regards to the ethical and legal requirements of practice; issues related to confidentiality; systems of record keeping;

(Continued)

(Continued)

the uniform code; policy on sickness and absence; emergency policies and procedures; break times and where to store their belongings? Are they invited out to social events or to join in with other informal activities such as book swaps, etc.? Most importantly, does this induction make them feel part of the team?

Once you have completed the above, consider if anything needs to be done differently to help students develop a sense of belonging and being part of the team.

There is a model answer to this activity at the end of the chapter.

Activity 3.5 focuses on the start of a student's placement. It is also important that the learning environment is safe and effective throughout the student's time with you. Gaining feedback from students about the range and quality of learning opportunities and responding to issues quickly and efficiently will ensure this is more robust. It may be that exceptional circumstances arise while a student is with you; for example, an outbreak of infection, a particularly unpredictable event or serious concerns raised following an inspection.

You may need to consider, along with the student, AEI and practice education team, whether it is appropriate for the student to remain or whether they should move to another area for a period of time. If it is the latter, then an action plan may need to be drawn up with the student which minimises the impact of this on their learning experience. Although these situations may not be very common, it is worth agreeing with the AEI how to best prepare for them. This would probably fall into the role of the person in your learning environment who is the named link to the AEI, sometimes referred to as a Learning Environment Manager. They may agree this process when completing the audit.

Keeping up to date on curriculum development – students should be very familiar with the content of their programme and which proficiencies they need to achieve while they are with you. It is important that you are also familiar with the programme and particularly the practice assessment documentation. One quick win is to attend update events which are usually delivered by the link lecturer from the AEI. These usually occur in the practice setting or online and often include an overview of the programme, the practice assessment documentation and opportunities for questions and answers. In addition, there are usually digital resources available including the full training plan for each cohort of students. Remember, if you would like to discuss a student's progression, you can contact their named academic assessor who should be clearly identified in their assessment documentation.

AEIs are continuously improving their education programmes and value the input and feedback from practice partners on new proposals and enhancements. It is a requirement of the NMC that practice partners have been consulted when a pro-gramme is being approved (by the NMC and university). This is a perfect opportunity for you to influence the education of the next generation of nurses and midwives. Your experience as a practitioner and practice supervisor/practice assessor is invalu-able and you may wish to talk to your link lecturer or academic link at your student's AEI about getting involved in such events.

Promoting professional behaviours – one of the most influential aspects of being a practice supervisor/practice assessor is developing the professional behaviours of students. The NMC guide on enabling professionalism outlines the five domains of individual professionalism (NMC, 2017b). These are learning and developing con-tinuously; being a role model for others; supporting appropriate service and care environments; enabling person-centred and evidence-informed practice; and leading professionally. These domains can be clearly articulated against your role. Probably the most relevant is 'being a role model for others', as the values you express and how you act in a range of situations are known to be powerful in shaping students' own values and behaviours. Being a role model includes the following behaviours and attributes: celebrating diversity; supporting colleagues and students; celebrating success (own and others); developing people to take on leadership roles and activities; and providing constructive feedback. In addition, another powerful attribute is the ability to accept and respond to constructive feedback and be 'open' to self-development. Chapter 5 has a detailed section on role modelling which you may find helpful to read before com-pleting Activity 3.6.

Scenario 3.3

Precious reads Jasper's Tweets and, after reflecting on them and discussing with Nell, confidently determines that he has not breached confidentiality. However, she does think that they can be interpreted as flippant and open to misinterpreta-tion. She feeds this back to him and he is genuinely surprised. Their conversation then turns to how difficult it can be to communicate complex information via social media. She is aware that the generations can relate differently to social media: she is Generation X and Jasper is Z. She reflects on their discussion and decides she will take more time to demonstrate how to convey complex and sensitive information to make this more explicit to him. She values Jasper's courage and commitment; these are key principles of the 6Cs (care, compassion, courage, commitment, communi-cation and competence), and she does not want to undermine his confidence but also thinks he needs to develop his skills around conveying complex information. Precious thinks back to one of her mentors and remembers what a brilliant role model she was and how much it made her want to work with students; she hopes that she can also be a good role model to Jasper.

(Continued)

(Continued)

Can you remember good role models that have supported your career and professional development? There are lots of studies which show the importance of role models for the socialisation of students into the profession. Students generally find clinical practitioners more relevant role models than their academic tutors and feel they are vital in helping them 'fit in' (Jack et al., 2017). Activity 3.6 further explores how the role modeller should model compassionate practice and leadership to enable the student to best learn from a situation.

Activity 3.6 Critical thinking

Looking at Scenario 3.3, what professional behaviours could Precious demonstrate to Jasper? What situations and learning opportunities should she try to make available to Jasper to enable him to develop in these areas? How can she make this learning more powerful for him? Jot down your thoughts in response to these three questions.

There is a model answer at the end of the chapter.

Chapter summary

As a result of reading this chapter and completing the activities, you should be familiar with the areas of educational governance and quality, as well as your role and responsibilities in assuring these. The recommendations of the Willis report highlighted inadequacies related to these areas and identified good practice. The chapter presented how AEIs and practice partners work together to ensure the recruitment of students who have the right skills and values to work in the NHS and wider healthcare sector. The NMC educational framework sets out the requirements for ensuring safe and effective learning environments, and the placement audit has been outlined. The chapter also considered how students should be supported to enable them to achieve, including those requiring reasonable adjustments. The chapter concluded by considering fitness to practise and professional behaviour issues. The importance of the practice supervisor and assessor being positive role models in upholding professional behaviours and ultimately protecting patients and the public was explained.

Activity answers

Activity 3.4: Decision-making (p52)

The following answer is not exhaustive but Precious should in the first instance gather a little more evidence. She could seek help from Nell in accessing the social media and exploring how it works, and further discussing the posts causing concern. She should view for herself the content of Jasper's posts and after viewing them make an assessment of the content and whether there are any breaches of confidentiality. Precious should get in touch with the link lecturer or other academic contact from Jasper's AEI and inform them of the situation. She can ask for information and guidance regarding using social media that the AEI provides, and make sure Jasper has a copy and understands it. She should then meet with Jasper in private and share the concerns with him. If she does not think there are any fitness to practise issues, she should feed back that other colleagues have raised concerns and also advise him to carefully consider the content of his posts. If she does have issues regarding fitness to practise, she should meet with the link lecturer or other academic contact from Jasper's AEI and agree with them how to progress this. She should ask Jasper to refrain from discussing his placement experiences on social media while they are investigating the concerns. Precious should inform her colleague Nell, who raised the concerns, that the situation is being managed, while protecting Jasper's confidentiality, and keep Jasper updated on any developments.

Activity 3.5: Team working (p53)

The evidence suggests that there are a number of things which help students to orientate to and feel part of the team, and therefore succeed on placement (Eick, Williamson and Heath, 2012). These include:

- acceptance in the workplace;
- feeling supported by the team;
- having a strong sense of nursing/midwifery as a profession;
- opportunity to discuss and make sense of difficult experiences.

Activity 3.6: Critical thinking (p56)

The following answer is not exhaustive but Precious could allow Jasper to observe her communicating complex and sensitive information to a client or family member. An example of this might be discussing the impact on the family of a dementia diagnosis. During this consultation she should convey empathy and allow time for reflection and clarification by the family and support them should they get upset. She should offer them the opportunity to ask questions and meet with her again if they wish to. Precious should check their understanding and give written information, including support organisations to them.

Precious can make this learning opportunity more powerful to Jasper by checking his understanding of her interventions and possible rationale for these. She could use self-disclosure to increase his self-awareness, for example that she felt sad when talking to the family. She could then link this back to Jasper's posts and how difficult it can be to communicate complex and sensitive information, especially via social media. Finally, she may suggest Jasper uses this situation as the basis of a reflective account. It is important she reassures Jasper that this is a learning opportunity, so he doesn't feel he has been chastised. This will make it more likely that he will ask for support in future, which ultimately enhances practice and protects patients.

Further reading

NMC (2019) *Guidance on Health and Character*. Available online at: **www.nmc.org.uk/registration/ joining-the-register/health-and-character**.

A helpful guide for employers, registration and practice and academic assessors and supervisors. This is a useful document to refer to as part of the revalidation process.

Royal College of Nursing (2018) Are *You Ready* for GDPR? London: RCN. Available online at: **www.rcn.org.uk/magazines/activate/2018/march/gdpr**.

Essential information and a useful toolkit produced by the RCN, specifically aimed at nurses.

Nursing and Midwifery Council (2019) *NMC Guidance on Using Social Media.* London: NMC. Available online at: **www.nmc.org.uk/globalassets/sitedocuments/nmc-publications/social-media-guidance.pdf**.

This helpful document applies social media use to the Code and outlines best practice when engaging with social media. We suggest you signpost every student to it at the start of their placement.

Nursing and Midwifery Council (2018) *NMC Enabling Professionalism.* London: NMC. Available online at: **www.nmc.org.uk/globalassets/sitedocuments/other-publications/enabling-professionalism.pdf**.

This is a great resource to help students to understand and develop professional behaviours.

Useful websites

Health Education England: values-based recruitment:

www.hee.nhs.uk/our-work/values-based-recruitment

Excellent resources to support values-based recruitment of students and employees.

NMC (2017) Revalidation:

http://revalidation.nmc.org.uk

Includes everything you need to know about the revalidation process.

Care Quality Commission:

www.cqc.org.uk

Find out more about the role and work of the CQC generally or your practice area/Trust.

Student empowerment

Standards Framework for Nursing and Midwifery Education. Part 1 of Realising Professionalism: Standards for Education and Training (NMC, 2018d)

This chapter will address the standard: **3: Student empowerment**.

3.1 Students are provided with a variety of learning opportunities and appropriate resources, which enable them to achieve proficiencies and programme outcomes and be capable of demonstrating the professional behaviours in the NMC Code (NMC, 2015).

3.2 Students are empowered and supported to become resilient, caring, reflective and lifelong learners who are capable of working in interprofessional and interagency teams.

The Code: Professional Standards of Practice and Behaviour for Nurses and Midwives (NMC, 2015)

This chapter most closely aligns with the following professional standards.

Practise effectively

7.1 use terms that people in your care, colleagues and the public can understand.

7.2 take reasonable steps to meet people's language and communication needs, providing, wherever possible, assistance to those who need help to communicate their own or other people's needs.

9.4 support students' and colleagues' learning to help them develop their professional competence and confidence.

11.1 only delegate tasks and duties that are within the other person's scope of competence, making sure that they fully understand your instructions.

11.2 make sure that everyone you delegate tasks to is adequately supervised and supported so they can provide safe and compassionate care.

(Continued)

(Continued)

11.3   confirm that the outcome of any task you have delegated to someone else meets the required standard.

Promote professionalism and trust

20.8   act as a role model of professional behaviour for students and newly qualified nurses and midwives to aspire to.

Chapter aims

After reading this chapter, you will be able to:

- understand what is meant by the terms student **empowerment** and **autonomy**;
- develop an understanding of key learning theories, styles and preferences;
- articulate the benefits to students of peer learning and interprofessional learning;
- reflect upon the impact of generational differences on learning preferences for students.

Introduction

This chapter starts by considering student empowerment as a prerequisite for effective learning and the importance of learning autonomy. We then consider the different approaches and models that help us to better understand how learning occurs and learning styles and preferences. The activities will help us to think about the relevance of these for different students we are working with. During this chapter we meet Sumatra, who is a practice supervisor, as she reflects upon the challenges that one of her students posed during a session, and she is thinking about the complexities involved in the process of learning. Peer and interprofessional learning are then introduced, and the relevance and some benefits of these approaches for students are identified. The chapter concludes by considering the implications of generational differences on students' learning.

Empowerment and learner autonomy

Empowerment and autonomy are terms that are often used together, sometimes interchangeably, and have become central components of health policy in relation to patient/client/service user care. But what do these terms mean when applied to learning and students? Learner autonomy describes self-directed and independent learning, where the student takes responsibility for their own learning requirements. Empowerment is a process required to enable the student to become an autonomous learner and continue to develop as they become increasingly independent (Allen, 2010). The NMC (2018b) states that the student should be at the centre of learning, empowered to take control of and responsibility for their own learning, and to self-direct their learning if safe and appropriate. Students should be provided with opportunities to develop their own practice and to work towards becoming independent, reflective and professional practitioners. This is critical in becoming a lifelong learner, which is a requirement for our professional registration.

How students take control and responsibility for their own learning is dependent upon several factors, for example the level of study, competence and confidence. However, to become empowered learners, they need to: have **access** to a range of learning opportunities; have a **say** in shaping opportunities; and have a **choice** for meaningful and purposeful engagement. Many educational theorists would argue that the most powerful learning only occurs through learner autonomy. For those of us supporting students' learning, we can have a huge impact on leading students to a more empowered state.

Here are some examples of how to support learner empowerment:

- **Create** a supervisory relationship with your student with an emphasis on student-initiated question-asking, rather than you asking all the questions. Ensure your student has access to you, colleagues and resources to help with answering their questions.
- **Ask** the student to talk about what they already know and skills they have gained. Encourage them to highlight areas they need to focus on during this learning opportunity. This might be identifying any gaps they have in their repertoire of skills or developing their practice around particular theory they have recently been introduced to.
- **Actively introduce and network** the student with other students, colleagues, resources who will be helpful in their learning journey.
- **Plan** activities that help the student to impact the wider environment they are working in; for example, handing over their care interventions to others and presenting case histories to others.
- **Emphasise** the uniqueness of the student's experiences and learning journey. Even previous negative experiences the student may disclose can be repackaged as learning opportunities.
- Ensure the **language** you use is appropriate for the student to be able to participate in relevant conversations. Be mindful of jargon and acronyms that are commonplace in your area, but might be unfamiliar to any newcomers.
- **Value** what your student has to say. Positively encourage participation in conversations involving care that your student is involved with. Create an atmosphere of mutual respect. Talking *at* the student, ignoring their thoughts and ideas, will disempower.

- If a student's ideas and thoughts don't correspond with yours or the necessary standards for practice, don't simply dismiss them. Instead, **encourage** the student to think about alternative ideas, introducing any relevant evidence, policy and guidelines supporting these. Provide time to discuss these developing ideas and thoughts.

Many of these examples are ideally best started in the induction stage when you first meet with your student. Induction is discussed in more detail in Chapter 2. This type of facilitative approach is also central to coaching, which is introduced in Chapter 6.

Andragogy and pedagogy

The students we encounter are adult learners. Towards the end of the twentieth century, educational theorists started to suggest that adults learn differently from children. In 1968 Malcolm Knowles proposed 'andragogy' was a better term for this process than '**pedagogy**'. The key difference between how adults and children learn is thought to be that adults are differently motivated to learn. While children often require extrinsic motivation and depend on instruction to be able to learn, Knowles found that adults were mostly self-directed and used their past life experiences in learning. Although the arguments no longer seem quite so clear for these differences, Knowles described how adult learners differ from child learners in the following ways (Taylor and Hamdy, 2013):

1. The need to know (why do I need to know this?)
2. The learners' self-concept (I am responsible for my own decisions)
3. The role of the learners' experiences (I have experiences which I value, and you should respect)
4. Readiness to learn (I need to learn because my circumstances are changing)
5. Orientation to learning (learning will help me deal with the situation in which I find myself)
6. Motivation (I learn because I want to).

Knowles (1980) suggests that because adults are self-directed, they should have a say in the content and process of their learning; adults have much life experience to draw from, so their learning should focus on adding to what they have already learned; as adults are looking for practical and applied learning, learning should be centred on solving problems instead of memorising content. These principles are helpful from curriculum design through to assessment strategies, not to mention during each and every learning encounter. They also complement student empowerment, putting the individual at the centre of the learning experience. Andragogy is further outlined in Table 4.1.

Scenario 4.1

Sumatra is a practice supervisor and is working with a number of students from different courses and year groups who have just started placements in her practice area. Recently she was teaching them about intravenous infusions. Sumatra had developed a session on anatomy with handouts, as well as facilitating a practical demonstration where the students had an opportunity to handle the related equipment. She noticed that one of the first-year students, Aisha, didn't seem to be learning this skill as well as the others. Sumatra has started to write a reflective entry in her journal about this:

I just couldn't think why Aisha didn't seem to understand what I was asking her to do. She wasn't even able to answer the questions in the quiz at the end of the session. The other students seemed to pick it up straight away and I was really pleased with them and told them so. I could see by the puzzled look on Aisha's face during the demonstration that she was struggling with this more than the others. When I asked her to demonstrate connecting the giving set to the bag of fluids, she opened the packaging incorrectly and dropped the giving set on the floor. She picked it up and started to attach it to the fluids without even commenting on what had happened. When I asked her if she thought it would be OK to do that for real, she just shrugged!

In Scenario 4.1 it seems that Sumatra has designed a learning activity without considering the different learning needs of the individual students attending the session. Although she has created a session that is relevant in content for the students, it will not be developing them as empowered or autonomous learners as it does not offer any opportunities for learning to be individualised.

Activity 4.1   Critical thinking

Using the examples of how to support learner autonomy and empowerment, and applying an andragogical approach with your students introduced earlier in this chapter, think about how Sumatra could have better designed the session.

There is a model answer for this activity at the end of the chapter.

Learning is generally defined as a process of an individual acquiring new knowledge, resulting in changes to their internal and external behaviours. Internally, learning might result in changes to an individual's way of thinking, their attitudes and their emotional responses. External changes are observable differences, for example how a student might undertake a practice task (Olson, 2015). Learning does not depend solely on the teacher or presentation of the knowledge. Instead, the student uses their own strengths and experience to enable learning to occur. You might have had a similar experience to Sumatra in Scenario 4.1 where a student hasn't seemed to have engaged in learning activities. Learning theories can help us to better understand how individuals absorb, process and retain knowledge.

Learning theories

How we learn is entirely individual and is influenced by cognitive, environmental and emotional factors. Our prior experiences as well as worldview affect how we learn or acquire new knowledge. There are many different theories about how we learn, although it is generally recognised that there are three main learning theories. These are behaviourist, cognitive constructivist and social constructivist learning theories, which are widely cited in educational text. In healthcare, two other theories are also used, namely connectivism and andragogy. Table 4.1 provides a summary of these learning theories and the teaching and learning strategies related to each approach (Aliakbari et al., 2015; Olson, 2015). Once you have read through the table, Activity 4.2 provides you with an opportunity to consider your personal views of knowledge and learning. Understanding learning theories and our own particular views about learning can help us to be more effective in supporting our students to learn as well as empowering them as autonomous learners (Olson, 2015).

Activity 4.2   Reflection

Take a few moments to think about your view of knowledge and how learning happens for you. Does one of the theories outlined in Table 4.1 best fit with your views? You might wish to make a note of this for your portfolio.

There is no model answer for this activity as it relates to your own views. However, if you would like to read more about theories of knowledge and learning and how learning happens, please access the further reading listed at the end of the chapter, in particular Aliakbari et al. (2015). This article outlines some commonly used theories in nursing and midwifery education, as well as the associated benefits and disadvantages.

The theories outlined in Table 4.1 have substantial differences in their views of knowledge and learning. The most significant difference is the theorists' views of how learning happens. One view is that knowledge is transmitted from teacher to student (behaviourist) while others view knowledge as something to be created within the individual (constructivists). This difference is because of the theorists' underlying philosophical thinking about the scope and nature of knowledge. Our underlying philosophical ideas will affect how we approach teaching and learning. Did you recognise which theory your views identified in Activity 4.2 most aligned with?

Learning theory	View of knowledge and learning	Associated learning theorists (major theorists are in bold)	Key principles of how learning happens	Motivations for learning	Helpful teaching and learning strategies
Behaviourism	*Knowledge and learning are behavioural responses to environmental stimuli.*	Ivan Pavlov, **B. F. Skinner,** Albert Bandura, John B. Watson, E.L. Thorndike	Learning is the acquisition of new behaviours based on environmental conditions. Humans and animals learn in the same way. Learning involves a behavioural change which is objectively observable. The teacher is *active* and the learner is *passive*.	The teacher uses stimuli to obtain a response, and rewards the learner once they have positively responded.	Compliment and praise good/ desired behaviours. Support the praise with evidence and examples wherever possible – for example, colleague or patient/ service user feedback. Utilise negative reinforcement. For example, if the student is displaying inappropriate professional behaviours, remove any opportunities for additional placement visits and activities until the desired behaviours are displayed.
Cognitive constructivism	*Knowledge and learning are processes of acquiring and storing information.*	**Jean Piaget,** William G. Perry, William Cobern, David A. Kolb, John Dewey	Mental structures (thus learning) are created from earlier structures, and not directly from environmental information. What happens *inside one's head* is more important than observable behaviours.	Motivation is largely intrinsic as it involves significant personal investment on the part of the learner. Learners become aware of the limitations in their existing knowledge and accept the need to add to or modify this existing knowledge.	Encourage the student to identify their own learning needs and how to pursue these (to *construct* learning). Encourage active participation in relevant activities. Identify the student's interests and build this into any learning experiences.

(Continued)

Table 4.1 (Continued)

Learning theory	View of knowledge and learning	Associated learning theorists (major theorists are in bold)	Key principles of how learning happens	Motivations for learning	Helpful teaching and learning strategies
			Knowledge is not passively transmitted from the environment to the learner. Instead the learner is *active* as a *maker of meaning*. Learning happens by applying previously acquired skills and knowledge to a new situation. This might involve adjusting previously acquired skills and knowledge, or accommodating new skills and knowledge, to better understand the situation.		Ask students to explain new material or experiences in their own words and assist them in assimilating this as they re-express the new ideas in their own language. Ask students to self-assess their own performance. Utilise problem-based-learning, reflection and concept mapping learning strategies. As a teacher, facilitate and guide learning as opposed to imparting lots of information.
Social constructivism	*All cognitive functions originate in, so must then be explained as products of, social interactions.* There is a variety of cognitive constructivism that places an increased emphasis on the collaborative nature of learning.	**Lev Vygotsky**	Learning is not just the assimilation and accommodation of new knowledge by learners, but the process by which learners are integrated into a wider *knowledge community*. Language and culture play essential roles in human intellectual development and in how humans perceive the world. These are social phenomena, thus knowledge is socially built (*co-constructed*).	Motivation is both extrinsic and intrinsic. Learners are partially motivated by the rewards provided by the wider knowledge community and as knowledge is constructed by the individual, they must have an internal drive to learn.	Facilitate group learning; encourage discussion based around a topic. With the student, identify a learning need and introduce them to the idea of networking with relevant individuals to help them learn about this. Follow up self-directed learning activities with discussions to further develop understanding, maybe presenting learning back to the wider team and giving encouraging comments.

Learning theory	View of knowledge and learning	Associated learning theorists (major theorists are in bold)	Key principles of how learning happens	Motivations for learning	Helpful teaching and learning strategies
			The learner's level of *actual* development is the level the learner has already reached, and where they are capable of solving problems independently. The learner's level of potential development is the level the learner is capable of reaching under the guidance of teachers or working in collaboration with peers. This is where learning takes place.		Use online resources that also offer online discussion forums. Facilitate a group debriefing at the end of a shift or after a particular incident. Utilise action learning sets, group work and peer learning strategies. As a teacher, facilitate and guide learning with and from relevant others, as opposed to imparting lots of information.
Connectivism	*In our digital society, the connections and connectiveness within networks lead to learning.* This is a variety of social constructivism and the work of Lev Vygotsky.	**Stephen Downes, George Siemens**	Learning occurs through connections within (digital) networks and by connecting to and growing personal networks. Learners learn through recognising and interpreting patterns. (Knowledge-based) decisions are based on rapidly altering foundations. New information is continually being acquired so there is a necessity to draw distinctions between important and unimportant information.	A learner's capacity to know more is more critical than what is currently known. A strong motivator is the diversity of the learner's networks, strength of ties and the context of their network.	Support the student in making new/maintaining relevant networking connections. An example might be connecting to other professionals in their field through workplace social media platforms. Support the student to improve their digital capabilities relevant to their developing practice. Signpost the student to evidence-based and research-informed practices.

(*Continued*)

Table 4.1 (Continued)

Learning theory	View of knowledge and learning	Associated learning theorists (major theorists are in bold)	Key principles of how learning happens	Motivations for learning	Helpful teaching and learning strategies
			Understanding of a particular area or field will happen more quickly if individuals are connected to networks, building evidence-based repositories. The potential to learn does not reside solely within humans and animals, but also within technologies.		Nurture the student's ability to see connections between ideas, and concepts as a core skill. Model how decisions are made within an ever-changing environment, and support the student in recognising quality data sources to help inform clinical decision-making.
Adult learning theory (andragogy)	*Adults learn differently to children and naturally tend to be more self-directed, internally motivated and ready to learn.*	**Malcolm Knowles**	Adults are at a mature developmental stage, thus they have a more secure *self-concept* than children. This enables them to take a greater part in directing their learning. Adults have a breadth of experiences to draw upon while they learn. Learning should therefore add to what is already known and build upon prior knowledge. Commonly, adults are involved in practical learning. Therefore learning should focus on/make explicit the links to issues related to practice.	Adults are internally motivated because: • many adults have reached a point in which they see the value of education and are ready to learn; • many adults return to learning for specific practical reasons, such as entering a new role.	Explain or provide the reasons and rationale for what is being taught. Any instruction should be linked and applied to practice examples and task-oriented instead of promoting memorising facts or knowledge. Teachers should take into account the wide range of different backgrounds of students, levels and learning styles to facilitate students to build on/link to existing knowledge and skills wherever possible. Adult students are self-directed, so any instruction should allow them to discover new knowledge for themselves. Utilise problem-based learning and self-directed approaches.

Learning theory	View of knowledge and learning	Associated learning theorists (major theorists are in bold)	Key principles of how learning happens	Motivations for learning	Helpful teaching and learning strategies
Hierarchy of needs	*Provides a model for how students are motivated to learn.*	**Abraham Maslow**	All students have basic needs which must be met for any learning to occur. Each level of need must be met for the student to move to the next level. The first level is physiological needs, then safety needs, then love and belonging, then esteem and then self-actualisation.	The teacher and student must strive to ensure each level of need is met in order for them to reach the next level.	First the necessities for life, i.e. food, water and shelter, are required. Students need to feel safe in the learning environment with no outside threats. Students need to feel professional belongingness with others in the learning environment, and that they 'fit in'. Students will feel confident in their ability to learn if they have good esteem, created through recognition and achievement. At the fifth level, self-actualisation becomes important and the student looks for ways to fulfil their personal potential for learning. At this level students will strive for certain learning goals and seek to achieve them.

Table 4.1   Summary of key learning theories and related teaching and learning strategies

Events beyond our control can also impact student learning. A recent example of this became apparent during the COVID-19 pandemic when many students (and staff) did not feel safe in the learning environment. This was reported in both the clinical and classroom environment, even though the recommended safety measures were in place. As Maslow's (1943) theory suggests, this resulted in them being unmotivated or unable to learn as they were preoccupied with safety concerns. For some students this resulted in them pausing their studies until they were able to feel this basic need was met, and only then were they able to resume learning.

Learning theories will have influenced educational practices in your clinical practice setting in some way. If we think about Sumatra's session in Scenario 4.1, she delivered some content that the students committed to memory and then were expected to complete an assessment (in the form of a quiz) of their learning at the end. When the students did well (desired behaviour) Sumatra rewarded them by giving them positive feedback as she was *really pleased with them and told them so*. We can see how this would fit with a behaviourist approach.

If Sumatra chooses to next ask Aisha to assess her own performance during that practical and then identify her learning needs before undertaking another assessment with this task, she could be utilising a constructivist approach. If she facilitates a group practical with all the students where they work on the same task and are encouraged to discuss their developing learning, it could be viewed as a social constructivist approach. From this example we can see how practice supervisors and assessors use approaches from learning theories in an integrated way to complement the particular learning experience. Educators are better equipped to support students if they have some understanding of these approaches.

Learning styles and preferences

The underlying principle of all learning styles, theories and frameworks is that individuals learn, but in different ways and at different levels. Different learning-style theories focus on how being aware of different learning styles can:

- Help students to understand which opportunities will best help them to learn. This can help to accelerate their learning, and make learning more enjoyable.
- Expand on the experiences students access. Going beyond activities linked to a student's *preferred* style will help them to become an *all-rounder*, which will maximise their learning opportunities.
- Support educators in planning opportunities which contain activities to suit students across all styles, encouraging maximum engagement.

There are many learning styles theories, frameworks and models available. They often involve using a questionnaire to identify an individual's distinct learning style or preference. Table 4.2 provides an overview of influential learning theories and models.

Model	Learners or learning-style categories	Overview
Myers-Briggs Type Indicator (MBTI) – developed by Katharine Cook Briggs and Isabel Briggs Myers (1975)	• Extroversion vs. introversion • Sensing vs. intuition • Thinking vs. feeling • Judging vs. perceiving	The MBTI asks questions about four sets of preferences, using opposing personality dichotomies, which result in one of 16 learning styles, or types. This tool is often used when establishing teams with complementary attributes. The first set is about how individuals gain energy, either from being with others or from alone-time and quiet reflection. The next establishes how individuals collect information, either gathering facts from the immediate environment or looking at the overall context looking for patterns. Thinking vs. feeling deals with decision-making, either looking for the logically correct solution or relying on emotions and values. The final set considers how individuals organise the environment and either prefer structure or for things to be open and flexible.
Experiential learning – developed by David Kolb (1984)	• Accommodators • Convergers • Divergers • Assimilators	Kolb's experiential learning theory states we learn continually and build particular strengths, which naturally lead to individual learning preferences, described as four learning styles. Accommodators are hands-on learners, preferring real experiences and enjoying new challenges. Convergers learn through problem-solving and technical tasks, and are less concerned with interpersonal aspects. Divergers use personal experiences and practical ideas from various sources and viewpoints. Assimilators learn best through ideas and concepts, rather than through people.
Mind styles – developed by Anthony Gregorc (1984)	• Concrete • Sequential	Gregorc considers the relationship between how we think and how we learn. This theory puts individuals on a spectrum between concrete and abstract thinking, and between sequential and random ordering of our thoughts. Concrete learning happens as our senses experience, while abstract learning deals with ideas. Sequential learners prefer information in a logical, linear way, while random learners prefer the unpredictable.

(Continued)

Table 4.2   (Continued)

Model	Learners or learning-style categories	Overview
Learning styles inventory – developed by Peter Honey and Alan Mumford (1986)	• Activist • Reflector • Theorist • Pragmatist	Honey and Mumford, building on the work of Kolb (1984), suggest individuals naturally identify with one or more of their identified learning styles. Activists are 'doers' and immerse themselves fully in new experiences. Reflectors are reviewers and learn from observing and collecting/analysing data to reach conclusions. Theorists, or concluders, learn by thinking through problems in a logical manner and value rationality and objectivity. Pragmatists are planners and learn through putting ideas, theories and techniques into practice.
VARK learning styles – developed by Neil Fleming (2001)	• Visual • Auditory Reading/writing • Kinaesthetic	Fleming suggests that visual learners prefer seeing (pictures, graphs, charts, diagrams, symbols, etc.). Auditory learners best learn through listening (lectures, discussions, tapes, etc.). Reading/writing learners prefer learning through using the written word (books, articles, notes, case studies, reflections etc.). Kinaesthetic learners prefer to learn through experience (practical tasks, hands-on projects, experiments, etc.).
Grasha-Riechmann Student Learning Styles Scale – developed by Anthony Grasha and Sheryl Riechmann (1996)	• Avoidant • Collaborative • Competitive • Dependent • Independent • Participant	This model focuses on student attitudes towards learning, learning activities, teachers and peers. Competitive learners feel they must compete with other students and enjoy activities where they can be judged for their abilities. Collaborative learners learn best by sharing ideas and talents, enjoying group work. Avoidant learners are unenthusiastic about learning content or participating and require support to motivate. Participant learners are good citizens and want to be involved wherever possible. Dependent learners learn only what is required, and will look to the teacher or peers for guidance on what to do and how to do it. Independent learners like to think for themselves, enjoy challenge and are confident in their learning abilities.

Table 4.2   Overview of influential learning theories and models

There are many websites where you can undertake a learning-styles questionnaire to help you identify your own learning style or preference. Familiarising yourself with the styles will help you to recognise traits and preferences in others around you. You might even ask your student about their preferred learning style. Table 4.3 explores how learning styles can be used to plan teaching activities.

Activity 4.3   Critical thinking

Take a few moments to think about your preferred learning style or preference. Which of the learning theories or models outlined in Table 4.2 do you find most useful? Do you identify with any of the learning-style categories associated with that model? Now think about some of the students you have worked with. Can you work out what their preferred learning styles might have been from their engagement with various learning activities? How might the learning styles affect how you worked together?

You might wish to make a note of this for your portfolio.

There is no model answer for this activity as it relates to your own style and experiences.

There are many models, theories and frameworks that attempt to identify an individual's preferred style, and you might have noted in Table 4.2 that there are overlaps and similarities between these. They all attempt to identify a preference rather than something that is fixed. Learning preference to one of the categories might be strong or weak and encompass a mixture of styles, rather than being totally captured in one of the boxes of the model. These can provide a useful guide to reflect on how individuals learn, rather than a label to confine and restrict a learner's abilities. Awareness of different styles can also help us to plan variation in our teaching and learning activities.

Learning styles are strengthened by individuals repeating particular learning strategies and tactics that they have found to work for them. Certain behaviours develop which then become habitual. Individuals may gravitate towards certain roles or career choices that fit with their preferred style. Honey and Mumford (2000) suggest that it is useful for students to be challenged with a range of activities to encourage them to be *all-rounders*. In Activity 4.3, did you strongly identify with any particular learning styles and could you recognise any of these traits in the students you have worked with? It is likely that we will be regularly supporting students who have a different style to our own. We might find our own style differs at different points of our career. Table 4.3 uses Honey and Mumford's learning styles to explore how we can use our awareness of learning preferences to plan a range of activities to not only engage our learners, but also encourage them to become learning all-rounders.

	Activists	Reflectors	Theorists	Pragmatists
Learn best from or actively look for activities where they have …	new experiences and challenges from which to learn short *here-and-now* tasks involving competitive team work and problem-solving approaches excitement, change and variety; *high-visibility* tasks such as chairing meetings, leading discussions and presentations; situations in which new ideas can be developed without constraints of policy and structure; opportunities for just *having a go*	permission or encouragement to watch/think/ponder on activities; time to think before acting, to assimilate before commenting; opportunities to carry out careful, detailed research; time to review their learning; time to produce carefully considered analyses and reports; help to exchange views with other people without danger, by prior agreement, within a structured learning experience; opportunity to reach a decision without pressure and tight deadlines	ideas offered which are part of a system, model, concept, theory or evidence base; time to explore methodically the associations and interrelationships between ideas, events and situations; opportunity to question and probe the basic methodology, assumptions or logic; opportunity to be intellectually stretched, e.g. by being asked to analyse and evaluate, then generalise; a part in structured situations with a clear purpose; visions presented, see interesting ideas and concepts, whether or not they are immediately relevant	been given an obvious link between the subject matter and a *real-life* problem; been shown techniques for doing things with obvious practical advantages; the chance to try out and practise techniques with coaching or feedback from a credible expert; a model they can emulate, or examples/anecdotes; been given techniques currently applicable to their own work; immediate opportunities to implement what they have learnt; time to concentrate on practical issues, such as drawing up action plans or giving tips to others
Learn least from or may avoid activities where they have …	a passive role (for example, lectures, instructions, reading); a role as observers; to assimilate, analyse and interpret lots of *messy* data; to work in a solitary way (for example, reading and writing alone)	felt *forced* into the limelight; felt they must act without time for planning; been asked for an instant reaction, or *off-the-cuff* thoughts; been given insufficient data on which to base a conclusion	no apparent context or purpose; to participate in situations emphasising emotions and feelings; to be involved in unstructured activities where ambiguity and uncertainty are high; been asked to act or decide without a basis in policy, principle or concept	been presented with learning that is not related to an immediate need they recognise; organisers of the learning who they think are distant from reality; no clear guidelines

	Activists	Reflectors	Theorists	Pragmatists
	statements that are *theoretical* – providing an explanation of cause; considerable repetition (for example, practising the same skill); precise instructions with little room for manoeuvre; a requirement to be thorough, and tie up loose ends	had to make shortcuts or do a superficial job, in the interests of expediency	been presented with a hotchpotch of alternative or contradictory techniques or methods without exploring any in depth; doubt that the subject matter is methodologically sound; a feeling of being out of tune with other participants, for example when they are with lots of activists	a feeling that people are going round in circles rather than getting to the point; political, organisational, managerial or personal obstacles to implementation; no apparent reward from the learning activity (for example, higher grades)
Examples of useful teaching activities include…	hands-on, practical experiences, demonstrations; simulation, role play; brainstorming, mapping group discussions, debate; puzzles, games, competitions	time out to process new information, skills etc.; paired or group discussions; debriefing after events; self-analysis, self-assessment and self-evaluation; multiple observation; opportunities to practise skills; feedback from others including peers, supervisors and patients/service users; regular meetings in a coaching, mentoring, clinical supervisor relationship	working through evidence base, research, pathways, guidelines models, statistics, quotes, stories, talking heads, patient feedback, background information, case notes, resource files; opportunity to apply theories	opportunities to put learning into practice in the real world; opportunities to try out new ideas, theories and techniques to see if they work; time to think about how to apply learning in reality; case studies, with real-life examples; problem-solving; paired or group discussion; regular meetings with practice supervisor

Table 4.3 Using Honey and Mumford's (2000) learning styles to plan teaching and learning activities

Activity 4.4   Critical thinking

Look at Scenario 4.1; it seems that Aisha's preferred learning style has not been accounted for in Sumatra's session. From your understanding of Honey and Mumford's (2000) learning styles presented earlier in this chapter:

1.   What might be Sumatra's preferred learning style?
2.   What might be Aisha's preferred learning style? What types of activities would best suit this style?

There is a model answer at the end of this chapter.

Although learning styles are widely used within healthcare education, there have been claims that learning-style measures are weak in reliability and validity, can be confusing to use and are based upon little evidence (Willingham et al., 2015). However, the focus of the criticism is on the effects of learning styles, not questioning their existence. Many studies focusing on nursing and midwifery students have shown the usefulness of teachers adapting their approaches to students' preferences. When teaching strategies are congruent to learning-style preferences, students are more motivated to learn, feel responsibility for their own learning, achieve higher grades and have greater satisfaction with their courses (Hallin, 2014). Understanding learning styles and related activities suited to different styles can therefore be incredibly helpful. When we are planning learning activities, the key is to ensure that we cover a range of activities that will help to engage and challenge our students.

Learning with peers

Students working together in a learning environment will be involved in similar experiences and will engage intellectually, emotionally and socially in *constructive conversation*. Learning occurs by talking and questioning each other's views to reach agreements or divides (Boud et al., 2014). This is something that occurs naturally. You might have noticed that if a student has a question, they will often intuitively ask another student. Students often feel safer going to a peer than a supervisor or assessor, whose experience or position might make them intimidating. A peer is closer to the student's own position and level of experience, so is more likely to have had similar questions and think in a similar way.

Peer learning is an educational approach available to practice supervisors, assessors and educators. It describes how students learn *with*, *from* and *about* each other, and is very current in the shift from teacher-focused to student-focused education. We can use this naturally occurring phenomenon by building in opportunities for peer learning. Peer learning is usually associated with **communities of practice (CoPs)** and the work of the social constructivist educational theorists. Instead of viewing learning as an individual process and as a result of teaching, peer learning assumes students construct their own understanding of what they need to learn. This is an essential component for students to become empowered in their learning and be autonomous learners. This approach is supported by the rise in the use of information technologies providing students with increased opportunities to learn and access networks. Activity 4.5 encourages you to think of peer learning opportunities in your clinical practice area.

Activity 4.5   Reflection

Can you think of a time when students in your practice area learnt together, or when you learnt with your peers? If so, did you notice any benefits from peer learning?

You might want to make a note of this in your portfolio.

There is a model answer at the end of this chapter.

Peer learning is a student-centred approach that can provide a richer student experience that effectively prepares the student for their professional roles as well as the diversity of the workplace. Peer learning in health professional education has gained significant momentum over recent years and has a strong evidence base supporting its efficacy. Studies have shown that students find it enjoyable and helpful to learning. In addition, peer learning can develop a student's skills in teaching and supervision, as well as in giving feedback (Boud et al., 2014). It has also been linked to **self-efficacy**, or the individual's belief in their ability to succeed; the creation of a feeling of responsibility towards one's own learning; and learner empowerment (Pålsson et al., 2017). You might have noted some of these benefits in Activity 4.5.

In Scenario 4.1, Sumatra could use peer learning to encourage the students to support each other with development of the new skill in her session. It is likely that some of the students in her group will have either seen or undertaken this skill previously, or have some knowledge to share relating to this. As supervisors and assessors, we can build in opportunities for our students to work together, encouraging peer learning wherever possible. As with most educational approaches, it works best when planned carefully and used appropriately. Peer learning should supplement time spent with a practice supervisor or assessor and never be used to replace that level of support.

Interprofessional learning

Interprofessional education (IPE) is defined as "two or more professions learning with, from and about each other to improve collaboration and quality of care" (Atkins, 2002). It remains a key component of healthcare policy, supported by governments, healthcare regulators and academic institutions. IPE is recognised as having the benefits for peer learning, as well as being a means to improve collaborative practice in the workplace. It adds an additional dimension to peer learning, by adding other professional lenses. As well as learning about one's own professional context, students learn about other professional contexts, to support a more joined-up and holistic approach to care. The World Health Organization (WHO) (2013) makes clear the link with IPE and collaborative practice in healthcare. In their report *Interprofessional collaborative practice in primary health care: nursing and midwifery perspectives* (WHO, 2013), they use six case studies in order to identify the enabling mechanisms and barriers to IPE. Activity 4.6 provides a summary of barriers to IPE and is useful for us to think about our own learning environments.

Activity 4.6 Evidence-based practice

Read this section adapted from *Interprofessional collaborative practice in primary health care: nursing and midwifery perspectives* (WHO, 2013). Think about whether any of these barriers are relevant in your clinical practice area.

Section 6.2 Summary of barriers to IPE

Professional cultures and stereotypes

In the process of establishing unique professional identities, healthcare professionals often overlook the value of teamwork and collaboration. Numerous studies have found evidence of professional cultures and stereotypes being adopted by health professionals. One of the most prevalent stereotypes among physicians is that they see themselves as the *leaders* and *decision-makers* whereas other healthcare professionals are considered to be the *team players*. Recognising that these stereotypes and attitudes become more entrenched with time, a number of scholars have emphasised the importance of addressing students' beliefs and assumptions early in their professional training.

Inconsistent use and different understandings of language

A wide range of terminology is used interchangeably to describe Collaborative Practice (CP); health professionals also have different understandings of what it means to *collaborate*. All the case studies showed that inconsistent use of language concerning CP resulted in inconsistency in reporting CP-related issues, which made data gathering and analysis more challenging.

Accreditation and curricula

Accreditation bodies for health professions determine what is included and what excluded from their curricula. Successful implementation of CP requires the inclusion of IPE in accreditation and registration requirements.

Shared vision

A shared vision was identified as a key enabler in the literature, helping to unify a team, and facilitating the achievement of its common goals. While all the programmes studied here define their goals, they do not label these as a shared vision. Only programme-specific goals were described, such as providing comprehensive HIV care, helping to fill existing gaps in healthcare systems, and promoting relationships between academics, the community and health services in primary healthcare, as well as goals on IPE for CP.

There is no model answer to this activity as it relates to your practice setting.

You might have identified particular barriers to IPE in your own practice setting in Activity 4.6, but what makes for a successful IPE learning environment?

Being aware of our own professional cultures and stereotypes; using consistent language; understanding how IPE fits with the curricula; and creating a shared vision are fundamental in the success of IPE. The literature also suggests that students get the greatest benefits from IPE when they direct the learning experiences, and opportunities are student-focused. The learning experience should be realistic and patient/client-centred as this provides the perfect learning environment for IPE (McDonough, 2016). However, IPE requires good facilitation. If we are working with students from two or more professional backgrounds, examples of learning experiences we could plan include: patient/client-centred case conferences; ward rounds; handovers; debriefing events after care episodes or specific events; group reflection; or action learning sets. In our roles as practice supervisors and assessors, we are ideally placed to ensure that IPE learning is developed and consolidated.

There are many ways in which we can develop our students to be empowered learners. Considering their individual learning preferences and styles as well as creating peer and interprofessional learning opportunities are all key. Another consideration we need to be mindful of is the 'generation effect' and the link with their potential learning preference.

Effects of 'generation' on learning

Different generations can be viewed as having unique cultures and characteristics, which in turn can shape their beliefs and expectations. This includes generational differences in approaches to learning. A report commissioned by Health Education England (HEE) called *Mind the Gap: Exploring the Needs of Early Career Nurses and Midwives in the Workplace* (Jones et al., 2015) outlines the different characteristics of each generation summarised in Table 4.4 (NHS Employers, 2017).

Generation Z are now entering undergraduate nursing and midwifery programmes and starting to become registrants. These will bring some different characteristics from those

Generation	'Baby boomers' born 1946–1964	'Generation X' born 1965–1980	'Generation Y' born 1981–1994	'Generation Z' born 1995–2010
Characteristics	Motivated and hardworking; define self-worth by their work and accomplishments	Practical self-starters, but work–life balance is important to them	Ambitious, with high career expectations; need mentorship and reassurance	Highly innovative, but will expect to be informed. Personal freedom is essential
Percentage of the NHS workforce	25%	44%	25%	6%
Attitude towards technology	Early Information Technology (IT) adopters	Digital immigrants	Digital natives	'Technoholics' – dependent on IT and little knowledge of alternatives
Communication preferences	Face to face, but telephone or email if necessary	Text messaging or email	Online and mobile (texting)	Facetime, Snapchat
Attitude towards career	Careers are defined and shaped by their employers	Loyal to their profession but not necessarily their employers	Working *with* organisations but not necessarily *for*	Career multitaskers, can switch easily between roles, more likely to have multiple careers

Table 4.4 Overview of characteristics of generations

of their practice supervisors and assessors. These students will have a tendency to prefer experiential learning and teaching methods, for example *how-to* videos of clinical skills, and working with passionate educators. Multiple resources must be quickly available to them to search and find answers. Seeing students using the internet and messaging constantly can be frustrating, but can be a useful learning resource. However, using the internet and messaging for personal use while in the workplace environment can create patient safety risks and should be discouraged. The NMC Code (2015) is useful to refer to if this becomes an issue with your students. The average Generation Z student will have an attention span of 8 seconds, which is much shorter than previous generations. They are likely to use the first information they get as they are looking for instant *answers*, so guidance on good and reliable evidence is required.

Generation Z students like learning in groups and social settings, as well as working independently at their own pace with resources tailored to their needs. They like teaching strategies that use technology and practical application, for example simulation and role play. As well as the differences in learning styles, the impact of these generational characteristics might be at play for Sumatra and her group of students in the Scenario. The key is offering choice wherever possible.

The potential impact of the generational differences is nicely summarised in the following extract from the summary of *Mind the Gap: Exploring the Needs of Early Career Nurses and Midwives in the Workplace* (Jones et al., 2015, p3), which helps us to think about the potential impact of the generational differences:

Through this work we have learnt that there are generational concepts that require consideration if we are to appropriately support individuals as they begin their professional careers. For the first time in history four different generations will be working together in the same employment environment. There are generational differences in values, expectations, perceptions and motivations in the current workforce and these are highly relevant in terms of staff education and engagement. Understanding differing motivational needs across these generations offers employers and education providers a real opportunity to better align support to meet individual needs and to improve recruitment and retention.

Chapter summary

This chapter has introduced you to the key concepts of student empowerment and autonomy. It has provided an overview of the literature around learning theories and learning styles. By completing the activities, you have considered how your preferred learning style might impact upon how you and your students learn. Through the chapter Scenario, we noted how understanding how our students learn can equip practice supervisors and practice assessors to individualise learning. Given the increased focus on interprofessional working in healthcare, we considered the benefits of peer and interprofessional learning as well as the links between student empowerment and collaborative practice. The chapter concluded by introducing another aspect that could influence student learning, namely the impact of *generation*.

Activity answers

Activity 4.1: Critical thinking (p63)

Using the examples of how to support learner autonomy and empowerment with your students introduced earlier in this chapter, Sumatra could:

- Provide an opportunity for students to develop the content of any sessions, arising from their needs. When the content is necessary or mandatory for the clinical area, make this clear and design the session with opportunities for student-initiated question-asking.

- Ask the students in the session to begin by talking about what they already know and the skills they have already gained relating to intravenous infusions, building on any previous experience. Ensure the students are aware that what is disclosed in the session is confidential, in case previous negative experiences are discussed. Encourage them to highlight areas they need to focus on during this learning opportunity.

- Provide opportunities in the session for students to work with other students, mixing levels of experience wherever possible.

- Plan activities that help the student to have impact, for example talking through their demonstration of the skill to Sumatra and other students.

- Introduce any jargon and acronyms that are related to this skill; encourage students to note any of these which are unfamiliar.

- Positively encourage participation, creating an atmosphere of mutual respect.
- Provide time for students to discuss the skill, introducing any relevant evidence, policy and guidelines supporting it.

Activity 4.4: Critical thinking (p76)

1. Sumatra might be an activist as the session she has designed has lots of activities designed for that preferred style.

2. We do not have enough detail to know exactly which learning style Aisha most identifies with. Aisha might require more time to reflect on the demonstration of the skill or to be able to see additional demonstrations (reflector). She might need to understand the underlying theory behind the skill, applying some of her related knowledge including fluid management and aseptic techniques, before being able to undertake the skill herself (theorist). Sumatra could use her understanding of learning styles to offer additional learning activities for Aisha. When she plans for future teaching sessions she should ensure that she covers a range of activities to engage students with different styles.

Activity 4.5: Reflection (p77)

There is no specific answer to this activity because these are your own personal reflections. However, you might have noted that peer learning is most effective when students are given an opportunity to get together to learn in small, collaborative groups. This might have been built into shift patterns or informally arranged. You can support peer learning by building into your students' work arrangements opportunities for them to meet with other students. You might have also noted that for peer learning to be effective, the group must have mutual respect, confidence and trust regarding one another. Each member must feel able to participate and have their voice heard. You can support peer learning by helping the setup of groups with introductions and ground rules.

You might have noted some of the following benefits:

- self-directed learning skills (associated with student autonomy and empowerment);
- motivated students;
- critical thinking and problem-solving skills;
- interpersonal and team-working skills;
- critical reflection skills;
- friendships and the social aspects of learning, tips and *survival skills* to help each other learn to nurse;
- peer teaching and assessment, especially found in clinical skill acquisition.

Further reading

Aliakbari, F, Parvin, N, Heidari, M and Haghani, F (2015) Learning theories application in nursing education. *Journal of Education and Health Promotion, 4.*

This article is a systematic review of the relevant literature, which combines learning theories research and nurse education. It outlines some commonly used theories as well as the associated benefits and disadvantages.

Davis, E and Richardson, S (2017) How peer facilitation can help nursing students develop their skills. *British Journal of Nursing, 26*(21): 1187–1191.

This article reports on the implementation of a peer facilitation scheme for pre-registration nurses. It offers an insight into how to implement this sort of scheme, as well as benefits that were noted.

Supervisors, assessors and educators

Standards Framework for Nursing and Midwifery Education. Part 1 of Realising Professionalism: Standards for Education and Training (NMC, 2018d)

This chapter will address the standard: **4: Educators and assessors**.

4.1 Theory and practice learning and assessment are facilitated effectively and objectively by an appropriately qualified and experienced professional with necessary expertise for their educational and assessor roles.

The Code: Professional Standards of Practice and Behaviour for Nurses and Midwives (NMC, 2015)

This chapter most closely aligns with the following professional standards.

Practise effectively

6.2 maintain the knowledge and skills you need for safe and effective practice.

8.1 respect the skills, expertise and contributions of your colleagues, referring matters to them when appropriate.

8.2 maintain effective communication with colleagues.

8.4 work with colleagues to evaluate the quality of your work and that of the team.

9.2 gather and reflect on feedback from a variety of sources, using it to improve your practice and performance.

9.4 support students' and colleagues' learning to help them develop their professional competence and confidence.

11.1 only delegate tasks and duties that are within the other person's scope of competence, making sure that they fully understand your instructions.

11.2 make sure that everyone you delegate tasks to is adequately supervised and supported so they can provide safe and compassionate care.

(Continued)

(Continued)

11.3 confirm that the outcome of any task you have delegated to someone else meets the required standard.

13.5 complete the necessary training before carrying out a new role.

Promote professionalism and trust

20.3 be aware at all times of how your behaviour can affect and influence the behaviour of other people.

20.8 act as a role model of professional behaviour for students and newly qualified nurses and midwives to aspire to.

25.2 support any staff you may be responsible for to follow the Code at all times. They must have the knowledge, skills and competence for safe practice; and understand how to raise any concerns linked to any circumstances where the Code has been, or could be, broken.

Chapter aims

After reading this chapter, you will be able to:

- understand the skills and attributes required to be a practice supervisor and practice assessor;
- recognise the purpose, benefits and principles of collaboratively supporting student learning in practice;
- articulate the benefits of using learning objectives and identifying student needs for maximising learning opportunities;
- develop an understanding of common teaching methods helpful for your role.

Introduction

Those who support, supervise and assess students must be suitably qualified, prepared and skilled, and receive the necessary support for their role (NMC, 2018d). In this chapter we meet Mike, who is a newly qualified registrant and is looking forward to supporting students in his practice area. He is planning to undertake the practice supervisor preparation required by his organisation. We are introduced to the skills and attributes required for this role, and consider the transferable skills and attributes Mike may already possess. We consider the benefits of working collaboratively to support students with their learning, as well as some of the principles involved in making this successful. Developing and using learning objectives and identifying students' needs are covered, as well as considering how these inform learning opportunities that are available. The chapter outlines common teaching methods used in clinical areas to support the student to apply theoretical knowledge to practice. The advantages and disadvantages associated with these are outlined, as well as the benefit of reflection to the practice supervisor/assessor.

Scenario 5.1

Mike is coming towards the end of his preceptorship period as a newly qualified nurse. He thoroughly enjoyed his time as a student nurse and although he found the initial transition to becoming a registered nurse difficult, he is enjoying his role on the ward he's currently working on. He has noticed that many of the students on his ward often request to work with him, and ask him for advice or information. Last week a third-year student called Lily started on his ward, and asked Mike if he would be her practice supervisor. She said to Mike that she found him to be very approachable and loved his enthusiasm for nursing. Mike was pleased to be asked, but knew that he had to decline. Unfortunately, he has not yet worked through the training package for practice supervisors that he needs to complete in preparation for the role in his organisation.

Mike enjoys working with students and has identified with his preceptor that he would like to do more of this. He thinks back to nurses who supervised and assessed him when he was a student and compares himself to how they were. He is anticipating that there will be a lot to learn and he might not be able to fulfil the role requirements. One of his colleagues has said to him that he will need years of experience before he can supervise students. Although Mike knows from the NMC education standards that this is not true, it has made him a little apprehensive. However, he plans to start working through the learning package, and has spoken with the educational lead in his organisation about this.

Preparation for becoming a practice supervisor and practice assessor

In Scenario 5.1, Mike is planning to undertake his practice supervisor training but has been told by a colleague that he needs more experience. He clearly is able to fulfil these roles once he has undertaken suitable preparation, supported by his organisation and AEI. It is a myth that the number of years a health professional has been in their role equates to how good they will be at supporting practice learning. Many students enjoy working with more experienced students or newly qualified registrants. Students probably feel that as these people have recently been in their position, they are better placed to understand their needs and how to support them.

The NMC (2018b) states that the practice supervisor can be *any registered health and social care professional* who is supporting and supervising learning in practice in line with their competence. In addition, practice assessors are NMC-registered nurses or midwives who have been suitably prepared and receive ongoing support to perform their role. More about these roles is detailed in Chapter 1. However, the NMC does not prescribe an NMC-approved preparation programme for either of these roles as it has done in the past. The preparation requirements for both of these roles are outlined in Table 5.1.

Approved Educational Institutions, together with practice learning partners, must ensure that practice supervisors/assessors:	**Preparation for practice supervisor role**	**Preparation for practice assessor role**
	receive ongoing support to prepare, reflect and develop for effective supervision and contribution to student learning and assessment	undertake preparation or evidence prior learning and experience that enables them to demonstrate achievement of the following minimum outcomes:
	have understanding of the proficiencies and programme outcomes they are supporting students to achieve	interpersonal communication skills, relevant to student learning and assessment
		conducting objective, evidence-based assessments of students
		providing constructive feedback to facilitate professional development in others
		knowledge of the assessment process and their role within it

Table 5.1 Preparation requirements for practice supervisor and practice assessor roles (NMC, 2018b)

The NMC (2018b) requirements for practice supervisor and practice assessor roles as outlined in Table 5.1 are a helpful starting point for us to consider our suitability for these roles. Further exploring the skills and attributes required for these roles can help us recognise transferable skills we already have as well as any development needs.

Skills and attributes required for the roles

There are a range of factors that influence student learning in practice. These include the quality of the supervisor–student relationship and the practice supervisor and/or practice assessor's skills and attributes. Supervisors and assessors need to develop and refine a set of skills and attributes to enable them to effectively undertake the role. Table 5.2 summarises the key skills and attributes required when supporting student nurses and midwives in the practice area (Eller et al., 2014; Robinson et al., 2012; Huybrecht et al., 2011; Chandan and Watts, 2012).

Skills	Attributes
Facilitative of learning, providing guidance	Positive attitude
Experienced and clinically competent	Passionate and inspirational
Able to give and receive feedback	Approachable, patient and enthusiastic
A positive role model	Mutually respectful and trusting
Good time management skills, and creates space and availability	Kind, caring, compassionate
A good communicator	Committed to supporting practice education
Reflective of own practice	Confidence in their professional identity

Table 5.2   Key skills and attributes required to support student nurses and midwives in the practice area

You will notice that many of the skills and attributes presented in Table 5.2 are required for your professional role, and therefore you already possess a number. However, you might need to further develop these to apply them to a different context; from patient application to student/learner. In Scenario 5.1, we can expect that Mike already has some of these skills and attributes; for example, Lily told Mike he was really approachable and loved his enthusiasm for nursing. As students have previously asked to work with Mike, we can see the importance students place on these sorts of attributes. A large-scale study of key components of an effective **mentoring** relationship (Eller et al., 2014) found that infectious enthusiasm and passion for the work was one of the most important factors students cited. It is likely that Mike's local learning package for these roles will reflect these attributes and range of skills. Activity 5.1 will help you identify your own skills and attributes as well as identifying any development needs.

Activity 5.1   Reflection

Consider the list of skills and attributes in Table 5.2 and if there are any others you feel are important in order to successfully support a range of students in your practice area. Next, reflect on this list and decide whether you already have these skills and attributes or whether you need to develop them further.

Consider also how you acquired these skills and attributes, as this might help you develop any new ones. It will be useful to make a note of these.

There is no correct answer to this activity, as it depends on your own experience and skills. However, at the end of this chapter there are suggestions as to how you might get feedback on your skills and attributes from others.

Students learn and develop their own skills, behaviours and attributes through observing their supervisors' behaviours, including communicating with patients, carers and other health professions; problem-solving; and decision-making strategies. Each practice learning encounter instils values and qualities in students that will shape how they professionally develop and work with students. Supervisors and assessors act as gatekeepers to the nursing and midwifery professions and develop a future workforce that is fit for practice and purpose. This means we have a responsibility for providing students with a quality learning environment to ensure that patient safety and quality standards are met. The Mid-Staffordshire NHS Foundation Trust public inquiry report (Francis, 2013) highlighted the significance of staff values and behaviours when maintaining the standards of patient care. The impact that your role can have on developing the future workforce and maintaining the highest standards of care cannot be underestimated.

A collaborative approach to student learning

For many years, students have been encouraged to work with the wider multi-disciplinary team to enhance their learning experience and have a greater understanding of the workforce. The NMC (2018a) states that students must "have opportunities to learn from a range of relevant people in practice learning environments, including service users, registered and nonregistered individuals, and other students as appropriate". A collaborative approach to student support in the practice area describes a team-based approach to support. Many clinical areas have used a team mentoring approach to overcome issues associated with shortages of registrants prepared to support students in practice. However, the responsibilities for support, supervision and assessment have, until recently, been with the named mentor (NMC, 2008). The *Standards for Student Supervision and Assessment* (NMC, 2018b) have radically updated this approach. They have set out new guidance based on findings from other relevant reports and to best fit with today's climate and context. The RCN (2017b) noted that there had been specific problems with the mentor role, which included the difficulties experienced by students and mentors when registrants do not wish to be mentors. Examples include the mentor qualification being linked with promotion opportunities for many registrants. In addition, placement opportunities were limited based on the numbers of mentors clinical areas had. The RCN (2017b) suggested that a team or collaborative approach to supporting learning in practice can develop **communities of practice** that don't just rely on individual relationships.

A community of practice is a model of situational learning, a term developed by Lave and Wenger (1991). It is based on collaboration among peers, where individuals work to a common purpose, defined by knowledge rather than task. Communities of practice can develop naturally because individuals share a common interest, or they can be created with the goal of gaining knowledge related to a specific field. Through the process of sharing information and experiences, the individuals within the *community* learn from each other, providing an opportunity to develop personally and professionally. Many clinical areas and teams work and function as communities of practice. It therefore makes sense for student practice supervision to be undertaken by the broader team, and not just the responsibility of a named individual. The NMC (2018c, p97) states:

Practice supervision enables students to learn and safely achieve proficiency and autonomy in their professional role. All NMC registered nurses and midwives are capable of supervising students, serving as role models for safe and effective practice. Students may be supervised by other registered health and social care professionals.

Potential challenges associated with a collaborative approach to student learning include: students missing out on learning opportunities; students feeling unsupported if they are not sure who has responsibility for their supervision on a particular shift; and difficulties adjusting to working and forming supportive relationships with different staff. To prevent these issues arising, supervisors need to allocate adequate time to discuss with the team students' progress at the end of shifts (Caldwell et al., 2008).

Even though there are some possible challenges to this approach, the benefits of working collaboratively to support student learning greatly outweigh these. Benefits of this approach include: ensuring that those who enjoy supervising students have an opportunity to do it; students learn from a diverse range of registrants; supervision is timely; and students gain networking skills and a better understanding of team roles. When others are able to contribute to the student's assessment decisions, the risk of bias is reduced. If they only ever work with one person, students might feel that they have had an unfair assessment decision due to difficulties with an individual relationship.

The move by the NMC away from individual mentors to a more collaborative approach to supporting students in practice is supported by evidence. A review of the literature relating to best practice in clinical midwifery student supervision models concluded that adopting a collaborative approach is beneficial to the clinical area and student experience (McKellar and Graham, 2017). It provides a democratic way of working and encourages shared leadership, allowing for learning to occur from all those involved. Although there have been few studies to show the impact of this approach on nursing and midwifery students to date, it is an approach widely used in other health professions. This approach signals that supporting students is *everyone's business*, echoed in the NMC Code (2015), which states: "Share your skills, knowledge and experience for the benefit of people receiving care and your colleagues". Activity 5.2 will help you to begin to identify colleagues in your area who support students.

Activity 5.2   Reflection

Think about the area where you work, how many colleagues you work with and what their professions are. Make a list and identify if they are registrants; their disciplines; whether they are non-registered practitioners; or maybe they are a new type of healthcare worker.

Now think more closely about your colleagues and consider their role and responsibilities with regards to supporting students. Who could support student learning in your practice area, and in what capacity? Consider these roles individually and identify both the unique and shared features.

There is no correct answer to this activity, as it depends on your own experience and skills. However, at the end of this chapter there are suggestions as to some of the roles you might have identified.

Principles involved in student support

From undertaking Activity 5.2 you will have identified colleagues with whom you will be working collaboratively to support student learning in your practice area. However, it is vital that one individual takes a lead role in organising the learning experience. This will be a colleague who has been prepared for the practice supervision/practice assessor role and might have prior mentoring experience. Studies have shown that when no one person takes a lead role, this results in a poorer learning experience for the student (McKellar and Graham, 2017). If in your practice area students will be working with a range of supervisors, they should be allocated a *lead* practice supervisor who co-ordinates the placement experience. Who undertakes this role will vary depending on where you work, but this individual might be responsible for all the students in your placement. They will be the students' 'go to' person, should they have any queries or concerns relating to the placement. Daily supervision of students can be delegated across the team, and students will work under the direct/indirect supervision of a practice supervisor who is "suitably prepared" (NMC, 2018b). All staff in the work area will contribute to students' learning experiences in some remit, and provide feedback to the supervisor/supervisory team. This feedback is also critical for the practice assessor who takes responsibility for student assessment.

For this to work successfully, all those involved in student practice learning should understand their role in this. Effective communication and information-sharing are central to the success of this.

The lead will need to consider how the placement is organised on a day-to-day basis and communicate this with the student, who needs to be aware from the start who will be involved. Your practice setting may have an area to make the teams visible, with photos and names displayed. In Scenario 5.1, when Mike completes his preparation to become a practice supervisor he is able to be part of the team supporting students in his workplace.

As a member of this team, transparency and communication of the student objectives are essential. Mike will need to familiarise himself with the programme of learning the student is on, as well as where they currently are in this programme. Objectives will then be planned relating to student contact with practice supervisors and practice assessors. Practice supervisors might adopt a coaching approach to working with the student. This involves planning in advance the types of experiences the student needs and how you can facilitate that. When Mike is working with his student, he will check with the student at the start of each shift what their objectives are. Mike can then ensure that his student has the learning opportunities to work towards these objectives, and consider who else might need to be involved. He also needs to plan how evidence of achievement will be obtained, ready for the student to share with their assessor at a later date. A method of communication should be established between the team and be accessible by all, including the student. In Mike's practice setting, the team use notes pages within the student's learning log to plan learning activities and provide feedback on progression. Being part of a larger support network for students has the additional benefit of supporting newly developing practice supervisors. Activity 5.3 will help you further consider factors involved in working collaboratively with others to support students' learning.

Activity 5.3 Evidence-based practice and research

Look through these considerations involved in adopting a collaborative approach to student support (adapted from Caldwell et al., 2008). Consider who has the responsibilities for the factors or issues to be considered in your workplace. Do you recognise your own responsibilities from this table? Does this highlight any additional actions that may be required for this approach to work in your practice area?

Considerations when adopting a collaborative approach to student support	Person/s responsible	Potential actions
Who will the team include? Do those individuals identified understand what's involved?	The person responsible for co-ordinating student support. This could be a clinical manager or education lead, for example.	Identify the team; ensure all members understand what is involved and their role in supporting the student. Facilitate any training as necessary.
Students require clear information about the approach to student support.	Those supporting induction activities. Practice supervisors will explain this at initial student meetings.	Provide written information for students to access about this approach before and during the placement.

(Continued)

(Continued)

Considerations when adopting a collaborative approach to student support	Person/s responsible	Potential actions
Students are allocated to work with suitably prepared practice supervisor/s and a practice assessor, and others.	Person responsible for co-ordinating student support.	Practice assessors will identify and facilitate other learning opportunities related to the student's learning needs.
Students need to be clear who can support their learning during each shift.	Allocated practice supervisor/s are responsible for delegating student supervision and teaching.	The student's rota should be planned to work with identified practice supervisors each day.
A practice assessor is responsible for assessment of the student, with contributions from the team.	An identified practice assessor identifies and facilitates opportunities to discuss the student's progress and competence. They will obtain feedback and evidence from the team members.	Time should be allocated for discussion to inform and enable robust assessment of students. A clear communication strategy should be in place. For example, a written system of communication can be used and accessed by all the team (and the student) if kept with the student's documentation.
The possibility of grievances being raised by students.	An identified team member, the practice supervisor or practice assessor deals with the grievance.	Deal with any issues in accordance with NHS and/or organisational policy.

There is no correct answer to this activity, as it depends on your own experience and skills. However, at the end of this chapter there are suggestions for next steps if you have identified factors or issues where no one in your workplace currently takes responsibility.

Identifying your role in supporting students, as well as the roles of others around you, is helpful to understand the rich learning context of your work area. Matching this to the student's own learning needs and objectives will help you organise the student's placements and plan relevant learning activities.

Learning objectives, needs and opportunities

The roadmap for building the knowledge, skills and behaviours required for registration should be transparent so that students and all those involved with supporting their learning can understand the start and end point and the steps in between. Learning objectives offer a common language and break learning into sizeable steps. They are also an essential tool to empower learners and situate them at the centre of their learning.

As learning objectives are commonly used within educational courses, students are generally familiar with them. They are statements describing the expected goal of the learning activity, or a description of the knowledge, skill or behaviour that will be acquired by the student as a result of the activity. Sometimes they are referred to as learning outcomes or learning goals. For some, the value of learning objectives is not fully recognised, as they are seen as being at odds with spontaneous learning opportunities. However, research shows that learning objectives improve student outcomes when teachers and students use them as a basis for planning activities, feedback conversations and assessments (Austin, 2018).

During conversations and meetings with your student, you can support the development of their learning objectives by ensuring that:

- a realistic number of learning objectives are set (these can always be added to during the placement if achieved);
- learning objectives take into account the level and experience of the student – they should be challenging yet achievable;
- a plan is developed of how they will be achieved, identifying potential learning opportunities, as well as how learning will be recorded.

Writing learning objectives as SMART objectives is helpful. A SMART objective is Specific, Measurable, Achievable, Realistic and Time-phased. The Department for Health and Human Services (2009) provides the following guidance for writing SMART objectives:

1. Specific:
    - Objectives should provide the *who* and *what* of learning activities.
    - Use only one action verb, since objectives with more than one verb imply that more than one activity or behaviour is being measured.
    - Avoid verbs that may have vague meanings to describe intended outcomes (e.g. understand or know) since it may prove difficult to measure them. Instead, use verbs that document action (e.g. 'At the end of the visit, the students will list three functions of the …').
    - Remember: the greater the specificity, the greater the measurability.

2. Measurable:

   - The focus is on *how much* learning is expected.
   - Objectives should quantify the amount of learning expected.
   - It is impossible to determine whether objectives have been met unless they can be measured.
   - The objective provides a reference point from which a change can clearly be measured.

3. Achievable:

   - Objectives should be attainable within a given timeframe and with available resources.

4. Realistic:

   - Objectives are most useful when they accurately address the scope of learning and steps that can be implemented within a specific timeframe.
   - Objectives that do not directly relate to the overall course outcomes will not help towards achieving these outcomes.

5. Time-phased:

   - Objectives should provide a timeframe indicating when the objective will be measured or a time by which the objective will be met.
   - Including a timeframe in the objectives helps in planning and evaluating the learning experience.

Activity 5.4   Critical thinking

The characters we met in Scenario 5.1 work together as part of a wider care team during a shift. Lily discusses at the start of the shift a learning objective she has previously developed with her practice supervisor. She explains to Mike that she would like to work on this objective today. The objective is: *I will plan and deliver care on my own to a group of patients.*

1. Is this a SMART objective?
2. Write a new objective for Lily based on her ideas and what you have learnt about SMART objectives.

There is a model answer to this activity at the end of the chapter.

Working with SMART learning objectives makes it easier for students to communicate what they are aiming to achieve as well as clearly articulating intentions to practice supervisors and assessors. Ensuring students' objectives are SMART from the start is an important step as this will help us provide support and feedback on learning and progress.

The term *learning needs* describes the gap between a student's current knowledge, skills and attitudes and the level they should have within a particular context. The context includes the stage of the course the student is at, as well as the speciality of the practice area they are working in. Regularly assessing a student's learning needs is therefore essential to help you plan relevant learning opportunities and activities. Students are encouraged to identify their own learning needs, and this activity is commonly built into practice assessment documentation. Students are commonly required to identify learning opportunities that are available; identify their own specific learning needs in relation to the placement; make a plan of how these are to be achieved; and record progress towards these outcomes.

Once students have identified learning objectives and needs, how these will be achieved requires consideration of learning opportunities. You can help your students identify different aspects of practice learning that will present the learning opportunities needed to develop knowledge, skills and behaviours included in the objectives. Students need to be provided with opportunities to connect existing knowledge with new learning. Placement offers a range of learning opportunities from formal ones, as described by your organisation in the initial placement setup and quality audit, through to informal opportunities that you can design and direct. Discussions with the multi-disciplinary team, shadowing colleagues and following a patient/service user as they have care interventions are all common opportunities. In fact, anything that extends knowledge, skills or behaviours and can contribute to developing competence can be a learning opportunity. However, it's not just about accessing opportunities, but about how students implement learning from these into their practice, or how it guides their development, that is important, especially in developing competence. Recording learning from opportunities is vital, to enable the student to establish the value and consolidate the learning. This could be through testimonies or reflections. Such evidence of learning is essential when it comes to making practice assessment decisions. Other common examples include:

- researching conditions, interventions, studying case notes;
- preparing for and presenting care at handovers;
- visiting related clinical areas;
- talking to carers and families regarding care experiences;
- attending courses within the organisation;
- broadening technical/equipment knowledge;
- reading specialist journals or textbooks.

There will be a breadth of learning opportunities for your particular practice area. Thinking about what learning opportunities are currently available or could potentially be available will help to prepare you for your role as a practice supervisor and/or assessor.

Activity 5.5   Leadership and management

Think about your learning needs in relation to your developing role in supporting students in practice. From this, write a minimum of one SMART learning objective for yourself. Remember that learning objectives offer a way of breaking down learning into sizeable steps. Once you have completed this task, list the potential learning opportunities in your work area and wider organisation, to help you achieve the outcome.

There is no correct answer to this activity, as it depends on your own experience and skills. However, you should talk with your colleagues about your answer. It would be useful to select colleagues who are already practice supervisors and assessors in your area, the Learning Environment Manager, the education lead, the link lecturer or your line manager. Whilst you are developing your new skills, it is important to network with others and find a role model who will help you achieve this. Referring back to your notes from Activity 5.2 might help you identify colleagues to help you with your developing skills.

Thinking of yourself as a learner with learning needs, as in Activity 5.5, can provide you with an opportunity to practise your skills in writing learning objectives. This will then help you to support students with writing learning objectives. An RCN toolkit published in 2017 provides guidance for mentors of nursing and midwifery students and includes a number of suggestions that should be considered both at the start of and during a placement (RCN, 2017a):

- Find out about the student's stage of training.
- Note any previous development needs and past mentor decisions.
- Ask about any specific learning objectives, competence and skills development required in the placement.
- Help the student to form achievable objectives.
- Introduce them to the placement learning opportunities.
- Ask if they need any additional support.
- Identify any specific learning needs/requirements for reasonable adjustments to be made.

Your role as a role model

Practice supervisors and assessors are role models for pre-registration students (NMC, 2018b; RCN, 2017b). Students will be observing and emulating the experienced registrants around them. Role modelling fits with the social learning theory proposed by Albert Bandura (1977, p22), who noted that learning would be "exceedingly laborious, not to mention hazardous, if people had to rely solely on the effects of their own actions to inform them what to do". Fortunately, most of our behaviour is learnt observationally, through role modelling.

Attributes linked to positive role models include being: approachable; friendly; calm; professional; highly motivated; up to date; competent; empathetic; and confidence-inspiring. We can see there are many overlaps with these attributes and the ones required for the practice supervisor/assessor roles listed earlier in this chapter. It is often the case that good role models are unaware that they are seen in this way. Students and other staff recognise these qualities and naturally drift to work with that individual wherever they can. In Scenario 5.1 we can imagine that Mike is an effective role model from some of the attributes Lily has fed back to him and he is often asked by students if they can work with him.

Learning from role models happens through our subconscious, whether learning was planned or unplanned. One of the fundamental benefits of role modelling is to help socialise students into the profession and working environment. From their first encounters in the work area, welcoming and including students and helping them to *belong* is critical to their development. This helps the student to establish the cultural norms. Role modelling helps students to learn the complex professional behaviours that are often difficult to describe. This important role is recognised in the NMC Code (2015), as point 20.8 expects all registrants to "act as a role model of professional behaviour for students and newly qualified nurses and midwives to aspire to".

Although the majority of experiences of role modelling are positive, students can potentially learn undesirable behaviours, and assume that the registrant is always correct and competent. Students might feel that they need to fit in and compromise their idealised concept of care delivery. Encouraging students to ask questions of their role models is therefore essential. Equipping students with critical thinking and problem-solving skills can help them to recognise good practice. Students have the opportunity to work with a number of supervisors and assessors; this exposes them to a variety of behaviours and encourages them to identify traits they wish to emulate in their practice as opposed to simply following what their official mentor does (Felstead and Springett, 2016).

Your role as a teacher

As well as experience and positive attitude, effective practice supervisors and practice assessors require additional knowledge and skills related to teaching and learning. Student nurses and midwives need to be prepared to be highly skilled and knowledgeable, to be self-directed and to work collaboratively and autonomously. As such, there are a range of student-centred teaching and learning methods to help to develop these attributes. Chapter 4 explores learning theories and preferred learning styles which empower students with their learning. In this chapter we build on this, and Table 5.3 outlines some of the common teaching methods used in clinical practice, as well as their advantages and disadvantages. Although these methods have differences, they share an adult learning approach in that as a teacher you are facilitative as opposed to instructive. It is important to note that no single best method exists. You might already be aware of your preferred methods when you are teaching students, peers or patients/service users/clients in your practice setting. However, as practice supervisors and practice assessors we are challenged to differentiate and adapt our teaching approach to meet individual students' learning needs and styles wherever possible.

Effective teaching methods can engage students in an active learning process and, if used well, students are likely to develop their knowledge and skill base. It is important for those involved in educating nurses and midwives to select appropriate teaching methods in order to deliver a high-quality educational experience. In addition, using a range of methods will add to student learning and engagement and develop your repertoire.

Reflective teaching practice

Practice supervisors and assessors will use a wide variety of methods and modes of delivery to facilitate active student learning. Reflective practice is a professional requirement as embedded in the NMC Code (2015) and standards for practice. Our patients/service users/clients wouldn't expect us to work as a nurse or midwife without having subject knowledge and skills and being familiar with best ways of practising. Equally, our students won't want to be supervised, assessed or taught by someone who doesn't know the subject or the best ways of teaching and learning. Reflective practice encourages us to understand students' needs in relation to our own abilities. Reflective teachers are more likely to be able to develop reflective students. Chapter 1 of this book introduces reflection and reflective practice in more detail. Activity 5.6 encourages you to reflect on an experience of teaching students or being taught as a student yourself.

Activity 5.6   Reflection

Reflect upon a recent teaching and learning experience, in particular the teaching method used. This could be one that you were involved in delivering to a student, colleague or patient/service user/client or you could reflect upon an experience where you were on the receiving end of the teaching and learning activity. The prompts are adapted from the NMC Revalidation Reflective Accounts Form (NMC, 2017a) and you may wish to use this activity towards your next NMC revalidation.

- What was the nature of the teaching and learning activity in your practice?
- What did you learn from the teaching and learning activity?
- How did you change or improve your practice as a result?

There is no correct answer to this activity, as it depends on your own experience and workplace. However, you might have noted a particular teaching method that you would like to explore further.

Read the section 'Teaching and Learning Approaches and Activities' in Chapter 5 of Gravells, A (2017) *Principles and Practices of Teaching and Training: A Guide for Teachers and Trainers in the FE and Skills Sector.* London: Learning Matters. This provides further insight into teaching methods.

Common teaching methods	What are these?	What are the advantages of this method?	What are the disadvantages of this method?
Lectures	This is one of the most basic teaching strategies, using a classroom/seminar room and a presentation. PowerPoint, Prezi and videos are commonly used to present information. Lectures tend to be less interactive and more teacher led. Online surveys can increase interaction.	Lectures can quickly provide a large amount of information to a large number of students; therefore they are efficient and cost-effective. They are useful to introduce new materials, complex content, models and frameworks. Can be delivered remotely, and recorded for future use.	They can be viewed as boring as they can put the student in a passive, information-receiving role. Students are exposed to information but are not given the opportunity to further process it. The teacher requires effective presentation skills for student engagement.
Seminars	A seminar is a group meeting, usually involving a presentation of some description from a teacher, then some related interactive work. The students should participate at least as actively as the teacher in a seminar.	There are similar advantages to those of a lecture except that seminar groups are smaller, with usually a maximum of 10 students recommended in a practice setting. In addition to introducing new information, the seminar then provides opportunity for deeper learning activities through student interaction and engagement with additional learning activities.	These often work best when students have undertaken some preparation work prior to the seminar, or have relevant experience to offer. They require facilitative skills from the teacher, and engaged, self-directed students.
Tutorials	These are usually a one-to-one session between a teacher and a student where both are equally active in the discussion and presentation of ideas. They are often used in universities and in traditional mentoring relationships in practice.	They are highly individualised for the student. They can be tailored to the student's needs, building on their previous experiences as well as clinical context. They can be useful to support assessment decisions in clinical practice areas. Especially helpful for meetings regarding progression. Tutorials don't require specific resources, and can be undertaken anywhere and at any time. Can be undertaken remotely.	They require facilitative skills from the teacher as well as a good understanding of the students' learning needs. The one-to-one nature of tutorials makes them resource intensive and potentially challenging for some individuals.

(Continued)

Table 5.3 (Continued)

Common teaching methods	What are these?	What are the advantages of this method?	What are the disadvantages of this method?
Simulation/ high-fidelity simulation	Simulation attempts to recreate a clinical scenario in an artificial setting. It has been a part of health professional education for decades as it mimics the care environment and allows for direct application of theoretical knowledge and skill demonstration, more than most other methods of teaching.	It provides experiences that help nurses and midwives develop clinical competence in a realistic and safe environment without the potential of harm to patients. This approach utilises the application and integration of knowledge, skills and professional behaviours, as well as critical thinking. It can broaden exposure to scenarios, and allows the student time to 'practise'. The NMC requires patient/service user, carer or community involvement in simulation activities where they are used to contribute to placement hours.	Simulation equipment is often expensive to buy/set up and maintain. Even in good simulation training events, it remains 'simulation' and not 'a 'real experience'. Simulation facilitators have to be well prepared in planning and running simulation events. A debriefing session is essential after any simulation to improve critical thinking and reasoning skills.
Role play	This is an interactive learning technique where students and teacher act out situations and scenarios. Helpful in experiencing the role of another or role expectations. The focus is not on acting but the actions of each 'player'.	Role play is often used to develop skills relating to communication, difficult conversations, professional behaviours and cultural sensitivity scenarios. They can be spontaneous, not requiring equipment or specific resources. Role play is useful to help practice assessors make decisions or clarify behaviours and judgements of a student.	Not everyone is comfortable with role playing and this might affect performance. In addition, some students might find it hard to take the scenarios seriously. Good facilitation skills are therefore required. A debriefing session at the end is required to improve critical thinking and reasoning skills.
Guided reflection/ reflective discussions	Reflection can provide a structure for students to make sense of learning experiences. This ensures that concepts and theories become embedded in practice.	Students can be facilitated to reflect during or immediately after practice experiences about what they have learnt. It is timely, and no additional resources are required. Students can critically appraise what has been experienced via their practice through reflection. This in turn will support improvement of their ongoing practice.	Reflecting critically and sharing this with others can be daunting for students. Some clinicians report that reflective discussion is more useful than written reflection, which can be time consuming. Also, reflective discussions are not always helpful if the teacher's assessment differs from the student's assessment of their practice.

Common teaching methods	What are these?	What are the advantages of this method?	What are the disadvantages of this method?
		Reflection can help students recognise how they are professionally developing and areas they are mastering.	Reflective practice is more difficult for some students' learning styles than others.
		When reflection involves others, it provides an opportunity to collaborate and share ideas about learning, changes and new ways of working.	However, all health professions have a requirement for reflective practice so working around some of the disadvantages is of benefit. The facilitator can discuss a requirement for open-mindedness and willingness to listen to others.
		Reflection also opens up an opportunity for open dialogue about a student's performance. Can be undertaken remotely, and set as a self-directed task.	
Care mapping	This is a technique to allow students to understand relationships between complex scenarios, cases and conditions, treatments and care options by creating a visual map. Mapping is logical, and flexible enough to be revised as further learning occurs.	Mapping enables students to visualise connections and links, building on ideas they already have, information they know already and experiences they have had, particularly with clinical cases and patient journeys. They also identify gaps in knowledge the student has, to help them further plan.	It is important for the teacher to provide feedback on maps to ensure students are not muddling the complex relationships.
		This technique helps students to analyse, evaluate and critically think about practice and theory. It can enable students to think holistically, understanding elements of care and the patient/service user/client experience. It can motivate students, offering learner autonomy.	This technique works well for visual learners, but may not be so effective for students with other learning styles.
Educational games/ gaming	Educational games are activities that have been specifically designed to help students learn. They could introduce information about certain conditions, treatments and interventions; or reinforce students' understanding.	Games can improve student knowledge through reinforcement of information. They are often used in addition to other methods, i.e. following presentation of material at a lecture.	Games take time and effort to plan and create. Even in their simplest form, they are resource intensive to develop, so consider the reusability of any game you create.
		Games encourage active learning and engagement. They can make the learning of difficult content more enjoyable.	

(Continued)

Table 5.3 (Continued)

Common teaching methods	What are these?	What are the advantages of this method?	What are the disadvantages of this method?
	Some games are designed to develop particular skills, for example medications management or leadership or management.	Games can be used for different levels of complexity. At one level this might be a matching game with labels and diagrams. Other games might involve strategy and encourage critical thinking skills. Games provide instant feedback. Games that can be played on mobile devices can make learning more interesting and connect students to a wider network of students.	If you use existing games, they could be expensive to purchase and for online games, there may be a subscription cost. Some critics of educational gaming suggest they reduce the student's attention span, which then impacts on other learning opportunities.
Problem-based learning (PBL)	This is a student-centred approach where students use 'triggers' from a case or scenario to acquire and apply information to the problem. Students learn through the experience of developing their own learning objectives, undertaking self-directed learning, then returning to the teacher to discuss and refine their acquired knowledge.	Teachers can use real patient scenarios, and require students to search for holistic answers. It's a useful method for complex information, for example clinical case management. This approach encourages self-directed learning; clinical judgement; real-world clinical problem-solving skills; working with others and across disciplines; and integration of theory and practice. The self-directed nature of PBL promotes the retention of learnt materials.	One common criticism of PBL is that students might not really know what is important for them to learn. This is especially relevant if they have little or no prior experience. PBL requires facilitative skills from the teacher as well as managing the discussion process and giving feedback on the learning. There is also a requirement of time needed for the student to undertake PBL.
Case studies	Case studies usually involve a description of a real-world situation involving a decision made and subsequent challenges and opportunities. Real clinical cases are commonly used, and clinical records and investigations are made accessible.	This is a useful approach in clinical practice as it bridges the gap between theory and practice. This is often an approach clinicians are very familiar with as case studies are reviewed regularly as continuing professional development activities or multi-disciplinary team meetings.	Students might identify issues that conflict with practice or the clinician's own decisions. This will need facilitation and debriefing to help the student make sense of practice or escalate concerns.

Common teaching methods	What are these?	What are the advantages of this method?	What are the disadvantages of this method?
	Case study findings are anonymised and presented to the teacher and/or others.	Case studies provide practice with recognising 'problems', articulating clinical practice decisions and evaluating interventions. This approach also supports students to be self-directed and think professionally whilst learning about practice. It requires no additional resources. Similarly to PBL, case studies develop collaborative skills as well as skills in organising oneself; researching; and presentation.	The case might have too narrow a focus, or if too complex may result in not enough depth about the condition being learnt by the student. There is also a requirement of time for the student to undertake a case study. Similarly to other self-directed methods, some students may struggle with what's expected of them with this approach.
'Bedside' teaching	This approach refers to clinical teaching in the presence of the *real* patient/service user/client. The learning interactions occur directly with the registrant, student and patient/service user/client.	This is a useful approach in clinical practice as it requires no additional resources and bridges the gap between theory and practice. This is often an approach clinicians are very familiar with. Students are provided with an opportunity to learn real-world clinical skills, clinical reasoning, communication, empathy and professionalism. It is particularly useful to teach a holistic picture of a condition, treatments and interventions. It should involve all three parties equally – each individual member brings their own value to the learning triad. The student brings condition-specific knowledge and the eagerness to learn; the tutor brings depth of knowledge, and willingness to help the student learn; and the patient brings relevant *real* clinical issues that allow the student to learn.	Bedside teaching needs to be student-focused, linked to the student's learning requirements and needs. There is a requirement to prepare the patient/service user/carer as to the learning experience. There needs to be a commitment to uninterrupted time for bedside teaching. The teacher needs to be prepared to deal with a number of different issues that might arise during the teaching and follow-up may be required after the teaching has finished.

Table 5.3 Common teaching methods used in clinical practice and their advantages and disadvantages

Using technology for teaching and learning

Most of us are increasingly using technology in our everyday lives, including learning activities. Perhaps in Activity 5.6 you reflected on a teaching session involving technology? Those of us supporting students should be aiming to understand how students use and interact with technology during their learning experiences. In addition, we need to be mindful of how tomorrow's registrants will engage with electronic health records (EHRs), wearable technologies, big data, data analytics and increased patient technological engagement. More than ever before, we need to support students to be open to technological advancements and challenges that do not yet exist.

Key findings from a research study of undergraduate students and their technology use by Brooks (2016) include:

- students have many devices they use to gather information;
- students have positive attitudes towards the use of technology for learning;
- students find the use of technology important for them to succeed;
- device ownership is higher among students than in the general population;
- the majority of students have a preference towards blended learning, utilising both online and face-to-face experiences.

Technologies that assist students in identifying individual strengths and weaknesses are particularly helpful for nurse and midwifery students. Also useful are smart devices and apps that can offer an opportunity for students to tailor resources to their learning needs as well as learning when they want to and at their own pace.

Technology-Enabled Care Services

Digital healthcare technologies are viewed as a means of addressing the big healthcare challenges of the 21st century and delivering the NHS Long Term Plan (NHS England, 2019). Following this, the Secretary of State for Health and Social Care commissioned the Topol Review (Health Education England, 2019), which explores how to prepare the healthcare workforce, through education and training, to deliver the digital future.

The use of digital technology is pervasive in people's everyday lives and recent figures suggest that 93 per cent of households in the UK have access to the internet, with 87 per cent of adults using the internet most days. Roughly 80 per cent of adults access the internet via a mobile phone, smartphone, laptop, tablet or handheld device. Importantly with regards to digital healthcare technology use, the gap between older and younger internet users is narrowing, with over 81 per cent of people aged over 75 years regularly accessing social media, messaging, online shopping and streaming services (Office for National Statistics, 2019). It is likely that these usage figures have increased following the COVID-19 pandemic, as more people have turned to digital technologies to keep connected during periods of isolation.

Technology-Enabled Care Services (TECS) describes a range of health and social care technologies such as telehealth, telecare, telemedicine, telecoaching and self-care apps. These have the potential to transform the way people engage in and control their own healthcare, empowering them to manage it in a way that is right for them. TECS are particularly used to help people manage chronic illness whilst remaining independent, as they allow for the remote exchange of information. This can be between a patient or service user and health or social care professional, and can assist in diagnosing or monitoring health status, such as blood pressure or promoting good health. TECS has the potential to address practitioner shortages and allows for people to be supported with their health and social care needs in their home environment (NHS England, 2015).

What does TECS look like in practice? You might already be using telehealth and video consultations to substitute face-to-face clinical appointments or monitoring your patients through specific apps. If not, it is highly likely that you will be doing so as the Topol Review predicted that within 20 years, 90 per cent of all jobs in the NHS will require some element of digital skills. Studies suggest that students are more likely to report they are digitally literate compared with their mentors in practice and are ready to engage with TECS as a learning opportunity (Brown et al., 2020). During the COVID-19 pandemic, remote consultations became the norm for many services and TECS were used to facilitate an effective learning experience for students. TECS placements were developed in many areas to provide learning opportunities for students who needed to work remotely, or to still be able to access placements as certain services were only delivered through TECS. These types of learning experiences are also viewed as a means of expanding placement capacity, as well as equipping students with digital skills required for the longer term.

To be able to supervise and assess students in this type of placement, you might recognise that you require support and training to have the competence, confidence and skills necessary to deliver TECS first. Health and social care organisations moving towards TECS recognise this and are committed to supporting clinicians to be digitally literate. As TECS evolve, and change the shape of services, we need to ensure students have access to these for their own learning experience as well as preparation of the future workforce.

Scenario 5.2

Mike has noticed that some students in his practice area appear to struggle with understanding the relevant anatomy and physiology related to his speciality. On occasions, he has directed them to books and articles he has found helpful for learning this. He asks around the students in his area about their preferences for accessing learning materials and finds out that the majority of students prefer to

(Continued)

(Continued)

look up anatomy and physiology information from internet sources. He reflects upon this and decides to research good sources of internet anatomy and physiology material linked to his practice speciality. He discovers an app that is free to use and interactive. As well as being informative and aimed at health professionals, it also includes interactive diagrams and video clips. There is also a short quiz to test learning, providing instant feedback. He now recommends that students download and use this app to support their anatomy and physiology learning.

Engaging with digital technologies to support your students' learning will help you to provide a good learning experience and meet the needs of diverse students. It will also help to develop the digital literacy of yourself and the students to meet the ambitions of the NHS Long Term Plan (NHS England, 2019).

Chapter summary

This chapter has introduced you to the key skills and attributes required to be a practice supervisor and/or a practice assessor. It has provided an overview of the purpose, benefits and principles of a collaborative approach to supporting student learning in practice. By completing the activities, you have considered the skills and attributes you bring to this role, as well as identifying colleagues involved in supporting students in your own practice setting. In addition, you have developed your skills in writing SMART objectives, as well as recognising learning needs and associated learning opportunities. Common teaching methods used in clinical practice have been introduced, as well as some advantages and disadvantages to these methods. Through the Scenario, we noted how every registrant has a part to play in supporting students' learning in practice.

Activity answers

Activity 5.1: Reflection (p87)

There is no correct answer to this activity, as it depends on your own experience and skills. However, you have probably noticed that you have many of these skills and attributes already. Thinking about how you have acquired these already will help you to work on any gaps. If you are not sure, seek feedback from your colleagues or students in your workplace. Reviewing your last appraisal feedback might also help.

Activity 5.2: Reflection (p90)

There is no correct answer to this activity, as it depends on your own experience and workplace. However, you have probably noticed that you have many different roles and registrants in your area who are impacting in some way on the students' learning experience. Maybe you have identified roles including: practice supervisors; practice assessors; learning environment managers; educational leads; link lecturers. These roles are introduced in Chapter 1 and you might want to refer to this chapter to further think about the roles you have listed from this activity. You might have listed others in your area that do not have a specific remit for supporting students, but who do this as part of their wider role. Roles will vary greatly between organisations. Your critical thinking in this activity might have resulted in you recognising that there is some overlap in the features of these roles.

Activity 5.3: Evidence-based practice and research (p91)

There is no correct answer to this activity, as it depends on your own experience and workplace. However, you may have noticed some factors or issues for consideration that you have no one responsible for in your workplace. It may be useful to talk about this with your colleagues, perhaps at a staff meeting, or with those in lead educational roles, for example a Learning Environment Manager. You might find it useful to read Chapter 3 of Ellis and Bach's book *Leadership, Management and Team Working in Nursing* (2015), published by Sage/Learning Matters.

Activity 5.4: Critical thinking (p94)

1. Lily's objective is not SMART.

2. A SMART version of Lily's objective would be: *by the end of the second week of placement, I will be able to plan and deliver all care required during the shift, to a bay of six patients under indirect supervision from a registrant.* This objective is SMART as it is specific in who is doing this and what it is; measurable; achievable in light of Lily's experience and level of training; realistic in terms of what she is required to do within her course; and has a timeframe to be achieved within the first two weeks of placement. Working with a SMART learning outcome makes it easier for Lily to communicate what she is doing, as well as for Mike to provide support and feedback on her learning and progress.

Further reading

'Teaching and Learning Approaches and Activities', Chapter 5 of Gravells, A (2017) *Principles and Practices of Teaching and Training: A Guide for Teachers and Trainers in the FE and Skills Sector.* London: Sage/Learning Matters.

This provides further insight into teaching methods and using technology for learning. It has many activities and examples to help you further develop skills in this area.

Chapter 3 of Ellis, P and Bach, S (2015) *Leadership, Management and Team Working in Nursing, Teaching Nursing Practice Series.* London: Sage/Learning Matters.

This book has some great chapters considering staff development and motivation, mentoring, supervising and creating a learning environment. In particular, Chapter 3 considers team working in detail, which is helpful in developing our collaborative approach to student support.

Chapter 6

Coaching models and approaches

Promote professionalism and trust

20.8 act as a role model of professional behaviour for students and newly qualified nurses and midwives to aspire to.

Chapter aims

After reading this chapter, you will be able to:

- define and describe coaching and its fit with the SSSA (NMC, 2018b);
- understand how to undertake a coaching conversation and use active listening;
- recognise some coaching models and articulate essential components of any coaching model;
- understand organisation coaching models and their uses;
- consider coaching attributes and their wider application.

Introduction

The SSSA (NMC, 2018b) state that "students are empowered to be proactive and to take responsibility for their learning", and in Chapter 4 we explored student empowerment in detail. Coaching is an approach to student support which is facilitative and encourages students to actively participate in their own learning. The focus of this chapter is on applying a coaching approach to student supervision and assessment.

To bring this approach 'to life' we meet Helen in this chapter, who is an experienced supervisor and assessor, and an aspiring coach. We explore what coaching is and how it differs from traditional mentoring roles. We review active listening skills and examine coaching conversations and tools to help structure these. We then look at some coaching models and how these can help us develop our coaching skills. We explore some organisational models of coaching, including Collaborative Learning in Practice (CLiP). The chapter concludes by considering coaching attributes and wider uses of coaching for your career.

Applying a coaching approach to the supervision and assessment of students

Coaching is an approach to working and interacting with others with the purpose of enhancing an individual's learning and development in a supportive way. The coach supports an individual ('coachee') to enable learning and personal growth. This learning can be varied, as the coach can help a coachee to develop not only their skills and capabilities but also their self-awareness, to better understand their future developmental requirements. Coaching can be a powerful approach because it is not only helpful for the 'here and now' learning, but can also better prepare the coachee for future learning. An effective coaching relationship can help coachees feel empowered to improve their abilities and effectiveness, thereby supporting students to be "proactive and to take responsibility for their learning" (NMC, 2018b).

The literature indicates the benefits of a workplace coaching approach to be: better engagement and overall workplace performance; improved sense of direction and focus; learner empowerment; increased motivation to learn; increased self-awareness; enhanced ability to communicate with and relate to/influence others; increased resourcefulness and resilience; and increased confidence (Bozer and Jones, 2018). It is clear that these outcomes are highly relevant to the NMC SSSA and therefore a coaching approach should be considered in relation to supporting and supervising our students. The RCN has helpful resources about coaching and its application to nursing. If you are interested in reading more, the link to these resources is at the end of the chapter.

Coaching and mentoring

Definitions of coaching commonly include principles such as it being a guided process which is time bound. The term coaching is often used interchangeably with mentoring and this can be confusing as there are substantial differences. Before we consider the differences, it is worth looking at the similarities and overlapping features. Both are focused on supporting an individual's development and involve one-to-one conversations where effective communication is paramount. In traditional definitions of mentoring there is an emphasis on the mentor using their own life experiences, skills and knowledge to support someone else to find their own solutions. The emphasis here is on the mentee finding *their own* solutions, which is the same for coaching. Both coaching and mentoring can contribute greatly to professional and career development, but in different ways. Coaching is generally time-limited, aimed at short-term goals and specific skill development, with an expectation of visible results. An example of coaching here is not from nursing or midwifery but boxing! In the film *Rocky III*, Apollo Creed acts as a coach to Rocky to help him develop a specific skillset for an upcoming fight. The relationship was time-limited (preparation for a specific fight) and focused on specific skills. For a coaching relationship, the coach and coachee may be matched because the coach may have a skillset the coachee desires/requires. This is the case with Creed and Rocky, as Creed had a quicker and more agile fighting style which Rocky needed to develop to win his next fight. The visible result of coaching here was skill enhancement, enabling Rocky to win.

In contrast to the coach/coachee relationship, mentors tend to focus on longer-term career development, providing continuous guidance and feedback for the mentee. Let us use another film example to illustrate this relationship: *The Karate Kid*. Here Mr Miyagi, the karate master, is a great example of an excellent mentor as he teaches the young Daniel not just karate, but valuable life lessons, and supports him in his journey to becoming a young man. The random tasks he sets of painting fences and waxing cars help develop essential life skills of patience and focus, before moving to fighting skills. Mr Miyagi adds value to Daniel's endeavours by passing on ideas and thoughts that aid his development.

Mentoring is less concerned with creating precise and focused behaviour change. Instead, its purpose is to help mentees build an appropriate larger picture that will illuminate their choices and significant decisions, such as future career choices. However, for nursing and midwifery registrants, the term mentor has historically been used to describe the person supporting the student learner in the practice area to achieve their competences, so might arguably fit more with the coaching definitions than mentoring. And, of course, until the launch of the SSSA in 2018, the mentor was also assessing student competence – which is different to both traditional **mentoring and coaching** definitions and principles. The SSSA offer the opportunity to utilise a coaching approach, given the assessment and supervision elements have been separated. Table 6.1 outlines the differences in coaching and traditional teaching/mentoring styles from the breadth of literature available on these areas. If you wish to refresh your understanding of mentoring, Chapter 1 addresses mentoring and its terminology in more detail.

Traditional mentoring/teaching style	Coaching style
Is directive	Is facilitative
The mentor provides answers and solutions	The coach asks questions and encourages the coachee to develop their own solutions
Conversations involve instructing and giving advice	Conversations involve asking questions which raise awareness, prompting, reflecting and listening
A longer-term relationship which is development driven	A shorter-term relationship which is task/performance driven
An informal structure: meetings take place when the mentee needs guidance, advice and support	More structured: meetings are scheduled around progression to goals
The focus is on the mentee's wider professional development	The focus is on the coachee's specific skill development
Typically, the mentor is more experienced in the mentee's profession	The coach does not have to have direct experience of the coachee's profession

Table 6.1 Differences in traditional teaching/mentoring styles and coaching styles

Coaching and counselling

We have looked at mentoring and coaching, but it is also helpful to consider the differences between coaching and counselling, as there is overlap between these definitions as well. The literature around these roles highlights that both might consider patterns of behaviour, and behaviour change mechanisms. However, there is an important distinction as coaching has its focus on the workplace, whereas counselling may focus on the whole spectrum of a person's life such as relationships, family dynamics and childhood. Also, coaches work with people who are generally functioning well but may need development in a specific area. This contrasts with counsellors or therapists, who work with people who are usually experiencing significant issues and more entrenched behaviours which may be influenced by negative thinking or past experiences (Piggot-Irvine and Biggs, 2020). When we are engaging in a coaching relationship with students, we need to be aware of boundaries, and not over-step these by encroaching on any personal and complex issues, should they arise during coaching sessions. Being able to recognise our role and personal limitations when it comes to supporting students is vital. Chapter 1 provides an overview of the roles involved in supporting students, and it is important to familiarise yourself with other specialist and expert support available, should you need to signpost students to any of these. Scenario 6.1 introduces Helen, an aspiring coach.

Scenario 6.1

Helen is an experienced nurse working in a GP practice in a semi-rural setting. As part of her role at the practice, she specialises in the management of respiratory conditions, and has undertaken additional training to enable her to manage her respiratory clinics and a complex caseload. Colleagues in the practice often refer respiratory patients to her and seek her advice.

Helen is an experienced mentor and undertakes both practice supervisor and practice assessor roles for a range of pre- and post-registration nursing students who come to the practice for a placement. She has recently undertaken a coaching course and is enthusiastic about its potential. Helen wants to develop her coaching skills further by using this style with her students. She regularly works with nursing students as well as students from other health professional backgrounds from the nearby university.

Andrew is a second-year nursing student who has been allocated a short placement with the GP practice. He is focusing on achieving part two of the proficiencies he needs to complete for his **summative assessment**. Helen is his practice supervisor for the placement and has been rostered to work with him as much as possible. His practice assessor is from another GP practice.

Ash is also undertaking a placement at this practice. He is a final-year paramedic student who is undertaking a week-long placement experience of non-urgent care settings. Although he hasn't formally been allocated to work with Helen, he has been advised to work a day with her to develop his respiratory care skills and knowledge, particularly with regards to patients who are not requiring urgent care but have chronic respiratory conditions.

Communication and coaching conversations

A recent, large-scale review of the literature highlighted the relationship between mentors' behaviours and student empowerment (Perry, Henderson and Grealish, 2018). This study highlighted the importance of effective communication and structured conversations on maximising student learning opportunities. The study also found that to encourage student empowerment and increase student self-efficacy during clinical practice, mentors should:

- Seek to be informed of students' learning objectives and abilities by providing a suitable time and place to listen to students discuss their abilities.
- Encourage students to take initiative and have control.
- Gradually allow students to take more responsibility and work independently.
- Empower students by expressing confidence in them and by facilitating their goal accomplishment.

These activities fit perfectly with a coaching approach and underpin most coaching models. The findings from this study provide us with a clear rationale for utilising coaching approaches when developing health and social care professionals and why coaching approaches are so relevant in the SSSA (NMC, 2018b). When coaching is used as an educational tool, it involves a well-defined set of goals and outcomes – which could be placement proficiencies and competencies. The coach is therefore usually an experienced practitioner, who then provides developmental support and non-judgemental feedback on the performance of a less experienced individual they are working with. In this context, a coach can help a coachee to develop a particular skill and provide evidence for future summative assessments.

Coaching, at its heart, involves a series of conversations that one person has with another. The coach intends to have conversations with the coachee that will benefit their learning needs and progress. Sometimes actions are required, for example the coach may demonstrate a skill for the coachee to then replicate, but at the very heart of the coaching approach is effective communication. Communication is a two-way process of sending and receiving information. In a coaching conversation, the coach presents their ideas in a way that the coachee can understand, and then listens to the coachee to understand how the message was received. Both parties need to be on the same wavelength. This might sound obvious, but we all have different values, experiences, backgrounds, expectations and opinions that affect how we filter and interpret incoming information. Active listening and checking how information has been received and understood is therefore a key part of any coaching conversation.

Communication and interpersonal skills are a critical part of any NMC-approved programme and emphasised in professional standard 7 of the Code (NMC, 2015). In Scenario 6.1, Helen has enhanced her communication and interpersonal skills by successfully completing a course in coaching. However, even without coaching training, she already has some essential coaching communication skills from her experience of working with students, patients and service users and it is likely you will have these too.

Scenario 6.2

Helen uses the NHS Improvement (2018) guide for active listening to help her prepare for her active listening during the upcoming coaching conversations. Here are her notes:

1. Define terms to promote clarity

Ensure I clarify technical terms and jargon. Encourage my coachee to identify his goals and learning needs clearly. Do not make assumptions about his prior learning. Use the terms used in the student's practice assessment document.

2. Repeat/paraphrase

Repeat back what the coachee is saying, using his words to enable me to check understanding.

3. Don't interrupt

Give my coachee space to talk freely as he shares his goals and what he wants from this coaching encounter. Use prompts or open-ended questions to encourage this.

4. Listen 'between the lines'

Try to 'hear' the coachee on all levels: his words, thoughts, feelings, assumptions, values, wishes and fears. Be alert to his body language; check he is not anxious and feels safe to be honest and open about his goals and any learning deficits.

5. Don't rush to fill silences

Be comfortable with silences as the coachee might be using them to reflect on what he is saying.

6. Feed back impressions

Check understanding from what the coachee is saying – summarise what he has said to ensure you are both on the same page with his goals and learning needs. To develop trust, show genuine interest, provide a safe environment and listen openly.

As a coach, as well as actively listening, Helen needs to plan the message she wants to convey and then ask her coachees questions which will help provide clarity and understanding. Summarising, achieved through effective questioning, helps check the listener's level of understanding. Feedback, both given and received, is the catalyst for making appropriate adjustments in the communication process to ensure you achieve mutual understanding, as you strive to identify and reach important goals with your student. Scenario 6.2 provides an example of Helen's active listening preparatory notes.

All coaching conversations should benefit the coachee, as they are focused on their individual learning and progress. The coach might use any combination of observation, open and closed questions, listening and feedback to create a dialogue that encourages self-insight for the student. The coachee should experience this as a focus on their learning, enabling them to develop a greater appreciation of their circumstances and any development needs. The coaching conversation should also provide an individually tailored plan, to meet any additional learning requirements or address any learning deficits. This facilitative approach can enable the coachee to develop their resilience, creativity in resolving issues and strategies to achieve future goals. Coaching conversations should be challenging whilst maintaining a safe and supportive environment. They should be thought-provoking and encourage the coachee to critically think about their performance and learning to maximise their professional potential.

The Scottish Social Services Council (SSSC, 2016) highlight the following core set of communication skills required when using a coaching approach:

- Attending to the other person involved in a coaching approach, building rapport with them and seeking to understand what is going on for them.
- Listening actively and carefully to the other person and paying attention to what they are saying and how they are saying it.
- Summarising or paraphrasing what the other person has said as a way of helping them reflect on their own situation, rather than giving advice or adding your own judgement.
- Using open questions which encourage the other person to say more, to reflect and understand more about their own situation.
- Being prepared to give honest, clear and specific feedback while making sure the relationship stays positive and open.

As highlighted earlier in this chapter, coaching is generally aimed at short-term goals and specific skill development which fits well with the practice supervisor role. The coaching relationship might last for part of a shift, one day or a whole placement. For Helen, Andrew and Ash, this is the case. Helen will use a coaching approach with Ash during the one day she will work with him, and also with Andrew for the duration of his placement. However long the relationship, feedback at a midpoint is essential to review progress and refocus if required. With Andrew, this can be planned in as a mid-point review meeting. For Ash, this might be a quick conversation partway through the day. Activity 6.1 offers you an opportunity to use a coaching approach and coaching conversations for your own development.

Activity 6.1   Leadership and management

Find someone to have a coaching conversation with, explaining to them that the purpose of this is for you to practise your coaching conversation skills. You could use the prompts in the NHS Improvement (2018) guide for active listening, introduced in Scenario 6.2, to help you prepare. Ask them to focus on a short-term goal or specific skill development, for the purpose of the coaching conversation practise. Given this may be your first attempt at a coaching conversation, it is advisable you ask the individual to focus on something small, rather than unwieldy or vague. Set a timeframe – maybe 15 minutes.

Next, reflect on the conversation: pay attention to how you started the conversation; how well you listened and used further prompts and open questions to explore the goal or skill. How did you manage the environment – privacy, distractions, etc? How much of the time did you talk? How much of the time did they talk? Were there any barriers preventing you from listening? What did you notice about your/their body language? At the end of the conversation, were you both clear in the agreed next steps or plan?

There is no model answer for this activity as it relates to your own experience.

We can draw from Activity 6.1 that the key skills for coaching are the ability to ask open questions and to listen effectively. Even though these are essential skills for our registrant roles, it is always helpful to practise these and fine-tune them for a coaching conversation. You might have noticed there were areas of the conversation that you felt went particularly well or maybe not so well. It might help you to develop your own coaching conversations checklist from this activity, to help you develop your skills in future conversations. Section 2.2, Core skills needed for a coaching approach by SSSC (2016), in the further reading recommended at the end of this chapter, is a helpful reminder of effective communication skills.

Coaching conversations may feel a little different to other types of conversations as they are goal-focused, and the coachee is central. Preparation is always helpful for coaching conversations, even though you are not the expert in the topic to be discussed. By preparation we mean thinking about open-ended and probing questions, as well as the structure of the conversation. Developing an understanding of coaching models and their strategies can help us navigate the conversation and this new way of working with students.

Introduction to coaching models

There are many coaching models and frameworks available to help us structure our coaching sessions or conversations. Models can help us implement a process by following a structure, until we become familiar and confident with the components.

These will not provide the answers for specific coaching situations – it's not about the content of the conversation – but instead provide us with a map and toolkit to be able to explore goals and concerns and facilitate the coachee into action. Coaching models offer a structure for the coaching conversation in micro, when you are in the moment of the coaching conversation, as well as in the overall coaching journey.

The models are not supposed to be prescriptive or rigid and the coachee's agenda should always be at the heart. Shelves in libraries are full of coaching resources, and you may be familiar with some already. Let us take a look at a few of the common coaching models and consider their commonalities. It is important to note that there are many other models that have been applied to the coaching relationship not introduced here. If you are interested in exploring coaching models further, please refer to the further reading section at the end of this chapter.

The GROW model

The GROW model (Whitmore, 2017) uses the GROW acronym to remind us of the coaching process and how to structure the coaching conversation: **G**oal setting, **R**eality checking, **O**ptions and **W**ill or **W**ay forward. As outlined earlier, the coach is not an expert in the coachee's situation, but instead facilitates them to navigate their journey by using these four prompts and stages. Each of the four stages are not necessarily discreet or sequential, and during the conversation they may merge. The important point to remember is that each stage has been covered by the end of the coaching conversation. Scenario 6.3 applies the GROW model to Helen's coaching conversation with Ash.

Scenario 6.3

Helen has arranged to meet with Andrew and Ash individually before they work with her. Andrew is starting a placement where he will be working with Helen most of the time. Ash will be spending just one day with her. She has chosen to use the GROW model to structure each coaching conversation and has prepared some questions. Here are her notes:

Goal setting: In this stage, the aim is to understand the goal or outcome that the coachee wants to cover in the learning encounter. I can ask: what would you like to get out of today/this placement; what is the most useful thing we can work on now; how does this fit with your placement outcomes? Goals should always be SMART (Specific, Measurable, Agreed, Realistic and Time-phased – this is explored further in Chapter 5).

Reality checking: In this stage, I facilitate the coachee to explore their feelings towards the goal, or any additional related facts. The coachee is encouraged to be

(Continued)

(Continued)

self-aware and have self-insight, as the reality of achieving the goal is examined. I can ask: how do you feel about …; how confident are you in your ability to do …; have you taken any steps towards … already?

Options: Once the reality about the agreed goal has been checked, the coachee needs to think about any actions, solutions or ideas that will help them to progress. The coachee is encouraged to develop these themselves and not be 'given' solutions by me. I can ask: what else could you do; what are the strengths/weaknesses of each of these options; are there any barriers which might stop you achieving …?

Will or Way forward: In this stage, I need to ensure the coachee is ready to act. This stage covers detail about any support needed, when things will happen, and any resources required. I can ask: what exactly are you going to do; what support do you need; when will you do …?

Activity 6.2   Reflection

Read Scenario 6.3 and the GROW questions Helen intends to ask Andrew and Ash in each of their coaching conversations. Think about how you could use the GROW model to structure a conversation with a student you have worked with; this might have been during a short or long placement.

Go through Helen's questions one step at a time and make these relevant to your coachee. Make a note of anything that you might find difficult to ask or any questions you might like to add and why.

There is no model answer for this activity as it relates to your own experience.

You have now had the opportunity to work through the stages of the GROW model. We now introduce a further step to this popular coaching model.

The TGROW model

This model adds an additional step, referred to as 'Topic', to the GROW model (Downey, 2016). This additional stage provides an opportunity to explore the topic the coachee wants to discuss if this is not already clear at the start of the coaching conversation. It is helpful at the start of a placement to provide the student with some direction and focus and ensure the learning outcomes for the placement are transparent. It might take place during the initial interview, and help the student and yourself as practice supervisor plan out learning opportunities to provide the relevant learning experiences identified.

Having a topic stage separate to the 'goal' stage helps to clarify the bigger picture before specific goals are set. You could ask: what would you like to achieve during this experience; what areas of your practice assessment documentation do you want to address; what is important to you to achieve during this time?

The OSKAR model

The OSKAR model is a five-stage model (Jackson and McKergow, 2006), again an acronym, which stands for Outcome, Scaling, Know-how, Affirm and Action, and Review. This coaching model has its origins in Solution-Focused (SF) approaches, originally designed for therapeutic use, but also applied widely in leadership and educational contexts. This is due to the pragmatic nature of SF approaches which can successfully and efficiently result in progress and behaviour change. Again, this model can provide structure to a coaching conversation and helpful prompts to ensure each stage is covered:

Outcome: In this first stage of the conversation, the emphasis is on encouraging the coachee to establish a commitment to the activity. Ascertain what they want to achieve through this learning encounter and what would be the perfect scenario for them. You could ask: what do you want from this session; how does this fit with longer-term outcomes; what would be the perfect outcome for you from this session?

Scaling: This stage refers to a way of helping the coachee establish a clear and quantifiable measure related to their goal. Scaling can help the coachee understand their learning deficits and progress, as well as identify further actions required. Coach and coachee can find this a helpful way to monitor progress and gain feedback. You could ask: on a scale of 1 to 10 where 1 represents … and 10 represents …, where are you on this scale in relation to this goal? Or on a scale of 1 to 10 where 1 represents having no experience and 10 represents having lots of experience of (proficiency), where are you on this scale?

Know-how: This stage is about helping the coachee establish what resources they have available to them to be able to meet their goal, including any skills, knowledge, experiences or attributes they already have which will help. The coachee is encouraged to critically think about any strengths. You could ask: have you done anything like this before; what prior experiences have you had that will help you with …; what did your previous supervisor feed back to you about …? What skills and knowledge do you have that might be helpful here?

Affirm and Action: This is an opportunity during the coaching conversation to focus on any positives, in relation to the goal. The coachee is encouraged to dwell on and reflect upon positive comments, and as a coach you can offer positive reinforcement. You could say: 'I am impressed by the knowledge you have about this subject and the preparation you've undertaken; from what you have said already that approach seems to work'. The Action stage involves the coachee being encouraged to articulate the next steps they will undertake in relation to the goal.

As coach, you might need to encourage these to be broken into sizeable steps if they appear overambitious or overwhelming. You can then use the Affirm feedback and questions following achievement of these 'mini goals'.

Review: This final stage of the model is an opportunity to review the coachee's progress against the planned goal. It is therefore likely to happen at the start of the next coaching conversation and offers an opportunity to refocus and redirect if required. You can ask: how did you do; what made that successful; what impact has that had on your assessment for this placement?

Egan's skilled helper model

This model was developed to help people in a range of helping relationships, to solve problems and develop opportunities (Egan, 2013). It involves three stages to help people move from inaction to action with an emphasis on empowerment. This model is further applied with a range of scenarios in Chapters 7 and 8 of this book. We have found it particularly helpful when supporting students with complex situations or goals, as it is concise and encourages thorough exploration of any issues at the start of the conversation. The three stages are:

Telling the story: In this stage the coachee is encouraged to tell their story and feel fully heard and acknowledged so they can begin to reflect on what is really going on. Your role here is to help them see the bigger picture and other perspectives to find a point from which to go forward. You could ask: how do you feel about …; are there other ways of looking at this; what is the best thing to work on now?

The preferred picture: This stage involves the coachee understanding what they really want from the learning encounter. This aims to generate energy and hope for the coachee to remove any potential barriers and see problems as opportunities to be ready to move into action. You can encourage brainstorming to facilitate imaginative thinking and then focus in on a goal by asking: what do you ideally want to happen; what exactly is your goal; what are the benefits of working on this goal?

Finding a way forward: This is the stage where the coachee is facilitated to think about how they will move towards the goals they have identified. This includes specific actions required, resources and anything that might support or hinder their efforts. You could ask: who/what might help; which ways are most likely to work for you; what will you do next?

Activity 6.3   Critical thinking

Looking through the coaching models introduced here, you might have noticed there are many similarities. All involve a method to move the coachee from where they are to where they want to be. You might already be doing this with students without even recognising you are using a coaching approach!

From your learning so far, what do you think are the essential components of any coaching model you can use? You can make a note of these for your own learning.

There is a model answer at the end of the chapter.

By completing Activity 6.3 and reviewing the model answer at the end of this chapter, you will have developed your understanding of the essential components of coaching. Now we will move on to look at how we can apply these coaching model components to all learning encounters and conversations.

Embedding coaching approaches into every learning encounter

Coaching models outlined earlier in this chapter are easier to manage when you have more than one encounter with a student, for example if you have been allocated to work with the student for the duration of a placement as a practice supervisor. But can we still use a coaching approach if time spent with the coachee is limited?

Like Helen, you might find a student works with you for a short period of time to develop their skill in one very specific area. Encouraging a structured approach to communicating goals and learning needs is part of any coaching conversation but becomes more critical when time and resources are limited. Using the student's practice assessment learning outcomes, and in particular SMART objectives, will be beneficial. These are explored in Chapter 5, so it may be useful to refresh your knowledge at this point if you need to.

Using a familiar communication tool to ensure communication is concise yet accurate can be particularly helpful when the student's learning encounter with you is brief. One commonly used communication tool you and your students are likely to be familiar with is SBAR. SBAR is an abbreviation for **S**ituation, **B**ackground, **A**ssessment and **R**ecommendation. It consists of standardised prompt questions in each of the four sections, to ensure that individuals share concise and focused information in a timely way. SBAR is commonly used as a tool for the communication of a patient's clinical condition, but it can be used to structure any form of communication to enable information to be transferred accurately and concisely between individuals (Institute for Innovation and Improvement, 2010). When working with a student for a very brief period you could use SBAR to structure communication of their immediate learning needs, to help you both focus when time is short. Table 6.2 outlines how SBAR can be used by a student in this way.

S (situation)	I am (name), on (course, year group)
	I am working towards (specific skill development/proficiency identified)
B (background)	I have (previous experience/exposure to the skill/proficiency identified)
	This could include any related experience, theoretical learning or simulated learning the student has undertaken.
A (assessment)	I want to learn to undertake (skill/proficiency identified) at (level of supervision required)
	This requires student self-assessment of learning needs related to the identified skill/proficiency. The student thinks critically of the learning encounter, combining any previous feedback/learning/evidence related to the skill/proficiency, considering any related formal assessment this is linked with.
R (recommendation)	I would like you to (expected practice supervisor/coach actions)
	Here the student articulates expectations of the practice supervisor/coach related to their identified learning needs.

Table 6.2   Using SBAR to structure communication of learning needs

Activity 6.4   Critical thinking

From your learning so far about coaching conversations, and reviewing the SBAR communication tool, imagine you are Ash, one of the students in the Scenarios, and use the SBAR tool to structure communication of your learning needs. You are hoping that your coach will write you a testimony based around one of your proficiencies, which will count towards your summative assessment. Remember: the aim of using this here is to articulate coachee learning needs quickly and concisely to the coach.

There is a model answer for this activity at the end of this chapter.

Activity 6.4 required you to put yourself in the position of a coachee to articulate your learning needs. This will be helpful if you do not have much time with your coachee. The first part of this chapter has focused on coaching conversation and models, and their application to individual supervisors and students. This was particularly helpful for Helen when she is working with Ash. But how can Helen use coaching to support all the students she is working with or who are in the practice at the same time? We will now look at how these approaches can be applied on a wider scale across a whole placement area or organisation.

Organisational coaching models

One of the ambitions of the NHS England (2019) Long Term Plan is to develop sustainable growth in the workforce and be able to 'scale up' the number of learners to meet the workforce requirements. During the COVID-19 pandemic, interest in nursing, midwifery and all health-related roles has increased, and to make the most of this opportunity, universities have increased student enrolments across courses nationally. If this 'scaling up' is to be met and any increase is to be sustainable, then placement capacity will need to increase, while maintaining the required quality and level of educational support. The Willis Commission (2012) asked for closer partnerships between higher education institutions and practice providers to ensure that student nurses receive the best preparation and support during their placement learning, with an emphasis on flexibility to meet challenging patient care demands. Organisational coaching models offer a different way of providing student supervision and have the potential to increase placement capacity. Let us now consider some of these.

Collaborative Learning in Practice (CLiP)

The Collaborative Learning in Practice (CLiP) model was developed in the UK by the University of East Anglia, and CLiP has been piloted and/or implemented in many areas since. We introduced CLiP in Chapter 1 of this book, as a model to organise student support in practice areas. Here we examine what is involved in CLiP and its coaching basis. You may be using CLiP already or be aware of areas in your organisation that are. In the CLiP model, coaching underpins the learning philosophy, and students are supported to take on greater responsibility for their learning. Importantly, the learning environment embraces a culture of valuing student-focused solutions to care (Lobo et al., 2014).

Lancashire Teaching Hospitals (LTHT, 2017) shared how they facilitate CLiP: 15–20 students are allocated to each placement area and separated into 'learning bays' with a coach who facilitates 1–3 students simultaneously to undertake holistic care of a group of patients. This includes undertaking essential skills, completing documentation, ward rounds and handover to the next shift. The coaches are overseen by over-arching coaches who maintain responsibility, complete the students' documentation and provide support. The learners complete a daily log of activities which are linked to a specific learning outcome such as understanding patient conditions, relative anatomy and physiology, prescribed medications and side effects. The students may visit other areas, including specialist bays within the placement, to follow their patient's journey whilst increasing their knowledge and experience. In CLiP, all healthcare professionals and care workers (not just nurses) may have input into students' support and education (Health Education England, 2017b).

The dedicated coaching role requires the coach to have no other clinical responsibilities during the shift, to be able to focus on supporting student learning. The coach will supervise a group of students of mixed experience, providing an opportunity for peer-coaching where appropriate. They observe, supervise and have coaching conversations that encourage the students to explain their practice and identify the learning. Coaches provide feedback to the students and their practice assessors for them to formulate an assessment of the students' performances. They provide written testimonies and might facilitate **formative assessment** opportunities. CLiP is defined by a more distributed approach to work-based learning, with educational roles shared between several qualified staff and with a group of learners.

Practice Learning at Northampton (PL@N)

Practice Learning at Northampton (PL@N) is a new model of practice learning for all student nurses at Northampton General Hospital that uses a coaching model, OSKAR (outlined earlier in the chapter), rather than the traditional mentoring model. This model is based on the CLiP model, but adapted by the organisation to suit its own context and requirements. PL@N is facilitated by registered nurses who have completed coaching training provided by the Trust. It uses the whole ward as a learning environment and aims to enhance the quality of the learning experience for each student year group. Third-year students lead the care for the group of patients they are allocated; second-year students initiate care and support; first-year students participate in care delivery with support from second- and third-year students.

The PL@N model encourages students to peer-support each other and share the responsibility of student practice learning. Groups of up to 16 patients within a ward are used for practice learning as PL@N bays. Three students of mixed experience are allocated several beds, supported by a coach for the duration of the shift. The shift coach is allocated each shift by the ward co-ordinator and will be a registered nurse who has undertaken OSKAR coaching training. It involves an 'hour of power' each shift which is reserved for studying, negotiated with the shift coach. This can be used to explore any relevant subject, for example disease pathology or patient management. As well as increasing placement capacity, PL@N has also been found to enhance the quality of students' experiences, making them feel more valued and part of the team (Ashworth, 2018).

Practice Education-Based Learning (PEBLs)

Practice Education-Based Learning (PEBLs) (Suffolk) is also based on the CLiP model but has been adapted and developed specifically for community hospitals and community care teams. This model puts the patient at the centre of learning activity, and then, like the layers of an onion, the students are closest to the care of the patient. Students are in small groups of up to three, preferably of mixed experience, or may be working individually with the coach if they are in the community setting. Each group of students is supported by a coach who is normally a registrant and has had coaching training. The next layer of support is offered by clinical educators and link lecturers who also take an active part in student learning. In the layer furthest away from the patient is the AEI and placement organisation, who also have a responsibility to support the students' practice learning experience.

This model is also based on the use of coaching to empower students, increase their leadership skills, problem-solving and critical thinking skills, and enable a smooth transition to the registered practitioner role (Health Education England, n.d.).

Collaborative Assessment & Learning Model (CALM)

The Collaborative Assessment & Learning Model (CALM) complements the SSSA (NMC, 2018b) with a collaborative team approach based on a coaching methodology to supporting learning in practice. Coaching is central, and coaching conversations emphasise the need to allow the student to explore and express their understanding, rather than supervisors being directive. This model aims to increase students' confidence and help them gain the ability to think critically and apply knowledge and skills to provide expert, evidence-based, direct nursing care.

Students are coached each day by a registered practitioner, utilising the expertise of non-registrants as required to meet learning needs. They are allocated patients to lead care for, dependent on their experience, prior learning and learning needs not limited to one bay. Peer learning participation for students is encouraged wherever possible. Electronic learning resources have been made available for students to use for self-directed learning, and they are encouraged to perform new clinical skills based on ability and supervision.

Coaches, and the wider practice team, have had training and access to resources regarding facilitating coaching conversations, and students are briefed on this approach during their inductions (Elliott, 2018).

> ## Activity 6.5   Leadership and management
>
> This chapter outlines the growing number of organisational coaching models; many of them require the supervisor to have undergone extra training on coaching. This activity requires you to find out what coaching activity and coaching training is available in your own organisation.
>
> Identify if there are any networks or communities of practice for colleagues who are using a coaching approach. Are there coaching buddy or support schemes for new coaches? If you are interested in developing your coaching skills further, you could enquire about opportunities to do this in your organisation. You might need to speak to colleagues in your practice area to help you with this activity.
>
> *There is no model answer to this activity as it relates to your own experience.*

Developing coaching attributes

Whether we are using coaching approaches in conversations, informally or in wider organisational approaches, the factors that impact positive coaching outcomes centre on the coach's facilitation skills and their attributes. Coaching literature referenced throughout this chapter indicates that these include the coach being acutely perceptive;

being diplomatic; having sound judgement; being confident; and having the ability to navigate conflict with integrity. You will probably have noted that the attributes required for this role are very similar to those required for the practice supervisor and practice assessor role, highlighted throughout this book. Therefore, as we develop our coaching skills, this in turn will develop our SSSA role development. Coaching and the SSSA (NMC, 2018b) really do complement each other.

As a way of developing these skills, you can ask the coachee for feedback on your coaching skills to determine areas for enhancement. Other evaluative factors include checking on progress made towards the coachee's goal, or whether any desired behaviour change has occurred. Students' placement evaluations will also help you evaluate the effectiveness of any coaching approaches you are using.

If we use coaching approaches and coaching conversations in our role working with students, it is essential we are self-aware of any related strengths and weaknesses. It is advisable for individuals working in a coaching role to have a coach themselves. It is often said that the best coaches have their own coaches, to help them fully reach their full coaching potential. You could ask your colleagues or line manager if there are any coaching schemes or networks within your own organisation.

You will find that coaching can be used for a wide range of other types of student and colleague circumstances. You could use your skills in artful questioning and appreciative inquiry to help others unlock their full potential to achieve their professional success with career coaching. You might be approached by individuals with a particular career coaching request, for example with leadership or educational development needs. It is likely that colleagues will start to look to you for support as your coaching skills develop, to help them to learn and grow as professionals. If you are interested in career coaching, the RCN have a range of online resources available. These include career coaching support with professional development decisions; registrant roles options; application and interview support; and managing careers around health and disability (www.rcn.org.uk/professional-development/your-career/coaching).

Chapter summary

After reading through this chapter and completing the activities, you will be able to understand how coaching and coaching approaches can be used for student supervision and assessment. Central to the philosophy of coaching is a belief in the potential of the coachee to improve their performance and develop their own solutions.

Key to coaching are coaching conversations that are safe, supportive and challenging; hopefully you will have developed your skills through the activities. These conversations will help to maximise the coachee's personal and professional potential, which in turn will impact the quality of patient care. You will have explored models to help us develop our coaching skills and ensure movement and progress. Through reflection on the coaching opportunities in your own organisation, you may have recognised that you would like a coach yourself. Whether during individual conversations or in more formal approaches to how student supervision is organised, we have learnt that coaching can truly empower students.

Activity answers

Activity 6.3: Critical thinking (p120)

In a large-scale literature review undertaken to compare coaching models and examine their relevance (Carey, Philippon and Cummings, 2011), the authors concluded that the critical components of coaching models are:

- Observation and feedback: observation of the coachee and then specific, constructive and timely feedback given by the coach.

- The coach–coachee relationship: one that allows for professional, honest and safe interaction.

- Clear problem identification and goal setting: undertaken at the start of coaching conversations to identify unambiguous and realistic goals.

- Problem-solving: the coach encourages the coachee to identify their own solutions.

- A transformational process: coaching provides a place for the coachee to improve their self-awareness and develop resilience.

- Stages or mechanisms by which the model achieves outcomes, which guide the process, ensuring all important aspects are addressed.

Activity 6.4: Critical thinking (p122)

S (situation)	I am Ash, a final-year paramedic student.
	I am working towards understanding non-urgent care settings during this placement.
	In particular, proficiencies relating to my HCPC Paramedic Standards of Proficiency: 'be able to draw on appropriate knowledge and skills to inform practice' in relation to respiratory examination and treatments.
B (background)	I have met these proficiencies in other placements relating to respiratory assessment and treatments: but in urgent care settings.
	I have accurately identified lung sounds during chest auscultation when assessing a patient's respiratory status during an acute scenario as well as during simulation. I have not heard lung sounds of patients with chronic conditions whilst they are 'well', or had an opportunity to explore treatment options for chronic respiratory conditions.

(Continued)

(Continued)

| A (assessment) | I would like to be able to identify lung sounds in patients with Chronic Obstructive Pulmonary Disease (COPD) and learn about their treatments. |
| R (recommendation) | I would like to observe you examining a patient with COPD, and for you to help me to identify the lung sounds during chest auscultation, as well as discussing treatment options. |

Further reading

Scottish Social Services Council (2016) *Coaching Learning Resource*. Available online at: **www.stepintoleadership.info/assets/pdf/SSSC%20Coaching%20Aug%2016%20master.pdf**.

Although this resource is aimed at individuals working in social care, it provides a great overview for anyone who wants to understand more about how a coaching approach could be helpful to them or develop their coaching skills.

Royal College of Nursing, Practice-based learning. Available online at: **www.rcn.org.uk/professional-development/practice-based-learning/professional-resources**.

This resource provides links to relevant publications and resources that support practice-based learning, as well as examples of innovations in supervision models from different areas of the UK.

Chapter 7

Curricula and assessment

Standards Framework for Nursing and Midwifery Education. Part 1 of Realising Professionalism: Standards for Education and Training (NMC, 2018d)

This chapter will address the standard: **5: Curricula and assessment**.

5.1 Curricula and assessments are designed, developed, delivered and evaluated to ensure that students achieve the proficiencies and outcomes for their approved programme.

The Code: Professional Standards of Practice and Behaviour for Nurses and Midwives (NMC, 2015)

This chapter most closely aligns with the following professional standards.

Prioritise people

1.2 make sure you deliver the fundamentals of care effectively.

1.3 avoid making assumptions and recognise diversity and individual choice.

2.6 recognise when people are anxious or in distress and respond compassionately and politely

Practise effectively

6.2 maintain the knowledge and skills you need for safe and effective practice.

7.1 use terms that people in your care, colleagues and the public can understand.

8.2 maintain effective communication with colleagues.

8.4 work with colleagues to evaluate the quality of your work and that of the team.

8.5 work with colleagues to preserve the safety of those receiving care.

8.6 share information to identify and reduce risk.

(Continued)

(Continued)

10.1   complete all records at the time or as soon as possible after an event, recording if the notes are written some time after the event.

11   be accountable for your decisions to delegate tasks and duties to other people (11.1–11.3).

Preserve safety

13.3   ask for help from a suitably qualified and experienced healthcare professional to carry out any action or procedure that is beyond the limits of your competence.

Promote professionalism and trust

20.8   act as a role model of professional behaviour for students and newly qualified nurses and midwives to aspire to.

25.2   support any staff you may be responsible for to follow the Code at all times. They must have the knowledge, skills and competence for safe practice; and understand how to raise any concerns linked to any circumstances where the Code has been, or could be, broken.

Chapter aims

After reading this chapter, you will be able to:

- recognise why you need to understand curricula to be able to support students with their progress;
- understand what is meant by assessment and competence, and key assessment methods;
- understand the purpose, benefits and principles of feedback;
- recognise when a student is 'in difficulty' and how to best support them;
- understand how to use the assessment process to manage a failing student and recognise when and where to seek support for your student and yourself.

Introduction

The NMC sets standards for programme curricula and assessments to make sure that students can achieve the outcomes required to practise safely and effectively, and most students will complete their placement without too many issues arising or causes for concern. Yasmeen is a student approaching the end of her second year and has a number of practice competencies still to achieve. In this chapter we meet her and her practice supervisor, Jan, at the start of Yasmeen's placement. This chapter begins by considering why Jan needs to understand the nature of Yasmeen's curricula to best be able to support her. Assessment of competence as a fundamental part of a student's curriculum is explored. We then identify common assessment methods and some of the quality issues associated with assessment. We consider the role others have to play in assessment decisions for our students. The purpose of feedback is then explored along with the implications it has for learning and progression.

Sometimes students do not achieve their practice assessment outcomes, and there will be a process to support them and you to record a failed outcome. In this chapter we examine issues around failing students, including indicators of failing and the processes involved to manage and support you and your student with this. Students might demonstrate behaviours we find professionally difficult yet are still able to progress through the programme as they meet their practice assessments. This sort of behaviour usually accounts for a student who is *in difficulty*. We meet Jez and his practice supervisor, who is concerned about his progress towards achieving his placement outcomes. We explore some of the signs and effects of students in difficulty, as well as failing students, and the process for managing this difficult situation. Supporting students in difficulty or who are failing presents a complex and challenging situation for practice assessors and practice supervisors.

Scenario 7.1

Yasmeen is a student nurse at the end of her second year on a community placement. On her first day she meets with her practice supervisor, Jan, to review her placement assessment documentation and set some objectives. She shows Jan the record of proficiencies that she is expected to achieve by the end of Year 2. Jan can see that Yasmeen has a number of gaps still to be 'signed off' as *safe practice* in the nursing procedures section, including: Nutrition and Hydration; Medicines Management; Assisting with Elimination; and Infection Prevention and Control. Yasmeen explains that on her previous placements, she has had little opportunity to be assessed on these clinical skills and that she would like to focus on these during this placement. She also explains that during her last placement she had to take a number of weeks' leave from the programme as she was the main carer for a close family member who has since died. Jan confides that she too has recently had a family bereavement and sympathises with Yasmeen.

Assessing proficiency

We regularly hear and use the terms *competencies* and *proficiencies* in healthcare practice, in relation to student assessments or the revalidation and pay awards process. The NMC uses these terms to describe the skills and ability to practise safely and effectively, without the need for supervision. It also details that proficiency must be consistently maintained throughout our careers (NMC, 2018a). Safety is the most important principle in the assessment of proficiency of registrant students and the standards reflect this by ensuring that students achieve a baseline level of proficiency at the point of entry to the register (NMC, 2018a, 2018e, 2019b). The NMC programme-specific standards inform the assessment requirements for the students you are working with, for example pre-registration nursing, nursing associates or midwifery, as well as re-registration return to practice and post-registration programmes.

How do we decide if a student is competent or proficient? There are two main approaches to considering this. The first focuses on tasks and skills and requires the direct observation of performance of these to evidence competence, an approach referred to as *behaviouristic*. It is sometimes criticised as focusing only on the task being assessed, rather than what the student might know, their underlying attitudes and knowledge and other attributes, and fails to understand the linkages of tasks to other aspects of care. The second approach considers proficiency or competence in broader clusters of abilities and is not so focused on a particular set of tasks. This approach is referred to as *holistic*, as competence is viewed as more than the sum of individual competencies. The criticisms of this approach are that individual proficiencies, evidenced through *tasks*, are easier to provide evidence towards and transferable to other areas (National Nursing Research Unit, 2009). Activity 7.1 provides you with an opportunity to reflect on which of these approaches is used in your practice setting.

Activity 7.1   Critical thinking

Think about how students' skills are assessed in your clinical practice. Which approach, behaviouristic or holistic, best describes how proficiency decisions are made?

There is a model answer for this activity at the end of this chapter.

Common components of practice learning assessments

Each of the NMC standards contains proficiencies which must be achieved by the end of the programme. The principle for assessment of proficiencies in each part is that the practice assessor completing the assessment should draw on a range of observed experiences in which the students demonstrate the required knowledge, skills, attitudes and values to achieve high-quality person-/family-centred care in an increasingly confident manner, ensuring all care is underpinned by effective communication skills. During each year or part of the programme, students are expected to engage at varying levels appropriate to their knowledge and understanding. At first students 'participate', then should be able to 'contribute', and by the end of the programme be able to 'demonstrate proficiency'. For example, the components of practice assessment for pre-registration nursing students include:

Professional Values: these reflect proficiency statements and are captured under the four sections of the Code (NMC, 2015). They are achieved by the end of each placement, and consistently throughout the programme.

Proficiencies: these reflect aspects of the seven platforms, communication and relationship management skills and nursing procedures (NMC, 2018a). They will be assessed in a range of placements but must be achieved at least once by the end of the year/part of the programme.

Episodes of Care: these are holistic assessments to facilitate student progress and must be achieved by the end of the placement/year/part (depending on the AEI).

Medicines Management: this assessment must be achieved by the end of the year/ part of the programme.

Patient/Service User/Carer Feedback: this is sought in relation to how the student cared for the person receiving care and contributes to overall student performance.

Recording Additional Experiences and Feedback: these are for the student to record reflections on their own learning, and for practice supervisors, peers and any others to record feedback.

Ongoing Achievement Record (OAR): this summarises overall achievements and provides a comprehensive record of student development and overall performance.

Achieving proficiency is an essential component of whether or not the student can progress to the next part, which usually occurs at the end of each year of the programme. As a practice assessor it is important for you to familiarise yourself with the practice assessment documentation used with your students, as well as their programme plans. Understanding the student's bigger programme as well as their experiences to date is critical in helping you to assess them accurately and fairly. You need to be aware of the stage or level they are at and where this particular placement learning experience fits with the wider programme. You can find details about the students' programme and curriculum from the academic staff from the student's AEI who are linked to your practice area. Activity 7.2 will help you to familiarise yourself with the documentation students bring to your practice area.

Activity 7.2   Decision-making

Identify and familiarise yourself with the practice assessment documentation that the students bring to your workplace. You might need to ask colleagues in your work area or from your AEI where you can access a copy of this type of documentation. If you have students from a number of AEIs accessing your workplace for placement, you need to be familiar with multiple

(Continued)

> (Continued)
>
> assessment documents. Although these might vary from institution to institution, they will all contain a common set of *proficiencies* required to be met for the student's programme, which will be mapped to the NMC standards (2018a, 2018e, 2019b).
>
> *There is a no model answer for this activity as it depends upon your own practice.*

Types of assessment

The practice assessment document is the key assessment tool you will use to assess a student registrant's proficiency, and we will now look at assessment in more detail. There are many forms of assessment, but the main types related to nursing and midwifery programmes are formative and summative assessments. **Formative assessment** refers to assessments for learning, to check on student comprehension, learning needs and learning progress. It provides a *diagnostic* opportunity to identify areas of strengths and weaknesses, from which action plans and learning objectives can be developed. It can also be used to monitor progress. In contrast, **summative assessment** refers to assessments of learning, which are usually formal, to measure learning outcomes or criteria at a specific point in the student's programme. This might be at the end of a placement, semester, part, year or end of the programme. Summative examples include written assignments and exams for theoretical learning assessments; and proficiencies and portfolios for practice learning assessments.

Let us now consider how these assessment types can be applied to practice learning. In Scenario 7.1, Jan sets Yasmeen formative assessments to assess her knowledge and skills about nutrition. She uses a series of questions, from which she might recommend some further reading and then observation of Yasmeen undertaking a nutrition assessment. Yasmeen will also complete a summative assessment in this placement which shows that she has achieved the required proficiencies, medicine management tests and that she has completed the required number of practice learning hours. Her practice assessment documentation will form part of the summative assessment to pass her second year of the programme, along with the theoretical summative assessments.

Assessment methods

In order to ensure that practitioners are competent, high-quality assessment strategies are needed. There are a variety of methods that can be used to assess a student practically and theoretically. Those traditionally associated with assessing theoretical knowledge include presentations, examinations, vivas and assignments. For assessing practice the assessment strategy should include assessment through observation of

Method	Description	Advantages	Disadvantages
Observation	This refers to observing the student undertake skills in practice. Assessors observe to see if the student performs properly. May be *continuous* (over a number of occasions) or *snap-shot* on a singular occasion.	Can be used to assess problem-solving abilities, communication skills, professional attitudes and behaviours if these are modelled during the skill performance. Plans, criteria or checklists used by the assessor during the observation can support the student's development if shared, and aid assessor objectivity. Often the most effective way to assess student practice, though best used when the assessor uses it with other methods, for example questioning.	Requires the relevant resources and opportunities to be available to undertake the observation of practice – this will need planning. Needs a systematic plan or set of criteria to help the assessor and student focus on what is being observed and assessed. Can cause the student to have *performance anxiety* and then to undertake the skill less proficiently than usual, referred to as the Hawthorne Effect. Being observed may cause the student to perform differently than usual.
Questioning	This refers to asking effective questions related to the practice learning. It enables students' thinking to be clarified, revised, affirmed and extended.	Can be used to assess previous knowledge or skills of the student. Can ascertain the student's ability to reason, critically think, problem-solve and synthesise ideas. Can provide feedback for how effective the learning for the student is/has been. It's quick, instant, cost-effective and can be undertaken anyplace/anytime.	Requires the assessor to use effective communication skills, understanding when to use closed and open-ended questions. Requires consideration of appropriate questions for the level the student is at. Bloom's taxonomy (Su and Osisek, 2011) is helpful for this, where the basic levels of remembering might require questions posed: how; who; why; what, etc. For deeper learning questions might be: *how might you do it differently?*
Quizzes	This refers to a short assessment that can gauge a student's retention and comprehension of a small amount of information. Might be verbal, written or online.	Can function throughout a placement as an informative feedback device allowing both the supervisor/assessor and the students to see where they are excelling or need more focus.	Developing a quiz requires an understanding of the curriculum and what the curriculum expects the student to know, as quizzes should be clearly aligned. Can be time consuming to develop.

(Continued)

Table 7.1 (Continued)

Method	Description	Advantages	Disadvantages
		Highly adaptable to different topics, for example: multiple-choice questions (useful for recall on guidelines and policy); true or false questions; short answer questions (useful when more understanding required); labelling diagrams (anatomy, equipment); filling in the blank/missing items (symptom management, care planning); matching items (drug interactions, etc.).	
Testimonies	This refers to a formal written statement about a student's performance, abilities, character or qualities.	Used to authenticate assessment decisions. A patient, service user or carer who has been on the receiving end of care from the student can be one of the most reliable sources of evidence. Equally, testimony from a colleague, another healthcare professional, can be a fantastic source of evidence for how your student performs when you are not with them, and in a different context.	The assessor must confirm that the information is authentic and current. The person providing the testimony should be informed as to how their testimony will be utilised. Guidance is needed as to how to undertake a testimony.
Simulation/ role play	Simulation/role play aims to replicate real patients/clients, scenarios or clinical tasks or to mirror real-life situations in clinical settings – with an emphasis on safety.	Useful for the development of technical-based skills required for clinical practice, in a safe environment. Enables assessment of infrequent events that the student might not have had the chance to encounter or experience. Can be set up at appropriate times and locations, and repeated as often as necessary. It can be undertaken in-situ with minimal resources. Feedback can be given to students immediately and allow them to understand exactly what went wrong/right and how they can improve.	Requires access to simulation equipment and other resources. Can be undertaken in amazingly high-technology simulation centres, which can be very expensive and require constant updates and maintenance. Not all students/situations are suitable for this. It takes effort and preparation to create meaningful experiences.

Method	Description	Advantages	Disadvantages
Self/peer assessment	Refers to the practice of self/peers grading or providing feedback on clinical skills and performance, based on guidelines or criteria provided by a supervisor/assessor.	Helps students to develop the ability to make judgements, which is both an academic and professional skill. Students gain insight into how peers tackle similar clinical problems. Students learn how to give and receive constructive criticism from peers. Can be an effective use of time and resources; supervisor/assessor acts as a facilitator.	May not be a reliable source of assessment evidence. Peers might not have the same understanding of the situation as the registrant. Students may not provide comprehensive feedback to each other. Students may show bias towards friends and avoid low marks for poor work as they might be concerned they may offend peers. Student may lack self-awareness to be able to do this.
Portfolio evidence/ reflective discussion	Refers to interpretation of an experience, identifying issues or questions that arise. Involves the creation of hypotheses regarding how to do things better, thereby challenging an individual's practice.	Portfolios allow students to review a broad range of practice and study in detail particular aspects of it. Can analyse strengths and deficiencies as well as reflect on and identify development needs. Through reflection, students learn to scrutinise their own performance and ask what went wrong as well as what went well. An essential professional skill.	Requires clear outcomes to keep reflections and portfolio entries focused. Requires understanding of reflective process; models can help this. Can take time to establish learning and provide an opportunity for feedback. May not be a reliable source of assessment evidence if the student is unable to use reflection or lacks self-awareness.

Table 7.1 Common methods of assessing clinical practice

care, simulation and evidence-based discussions. The NMC requires most practice assessment to be undertaken through direct observation of practice. Simulation may occur where opportunities in practice are limited. Other examples of evidence towards a proficiency decision include: **Observed Structured Clinical Examinations (OSCEs)**; testimony from others (including service users and carers); student self-assessment; written portfolio of evidence; active participation; interactive reflective discussion; learning contracts; guided study; interviews; peer evaluation; collection of data; case studies; and team feedback. Common methods of assessing clinical practice are further outlined in Table 7.1, along with associated advantages and disadvantages.

Assessment quality

A large-scale review of the literature relating to the assessment process of student nurses' and midwives' clinical practice found that it often lacks consistency, varies in quality and is open to the subjective bias of the assessor (Helminen et al., 2016). Clinical assessment commonly relies on observation of the performance of a student by another individual or *observer*, which runs the risk of observer **bias**. This describes the idea that there is a tendency for an observer to observe what they are expecting or wanting to see. When observing a student, the supervisor or assessor might have some prior knowledge or subjective feelings about the student that might affect their judgements. In Scenario 7.1, Jan and Yasmeen will have spent lots of time together during Yasmeen's placement. They might have spoken socially as they share long car journeys between their case visits and discovered they share some similar interests. When Jan is assessing Yasmeen's clinical skills, it is possible that she might not be able to objectively do this.

The NMC *Standards for Student Supervision and Assessment* (NMC, 2018b) clearly separate practice learning and supervision from formal independent assessment in an attempt to reduce bias. There is no longer a mentor model, where one person was responsible for all aspects of practice learning, supervision and assessment. Instead there are the two distinct roles of practice supervisor and practice assessor. Practice supervisors work with students on a regular basis. The practice assessor will not work with their allocated student on a day-to-day basis, but will have the overall responsibility for their assessment. If we apply these standards to Scenario 7.1, a colleague of Jan's will be assigned to be Yasmeen's practice assessor and they will be responsible for assessing Yasmeen, taking into account feedback from Jan, service users and peers as well as any reflections, thereby reducing observer bias.

Healthcare programmes usually include set assessments at key stages of the programme as well as continuous assessment throughout the programme. Continuous assessment aims to measure competence at varying points in time rather than at one key point. Assessment at key stages is to decide if the student is able to progress to the next stage of the programme, for example progressing into the next year.

With any assessments, two issues are important: how and what is being measured. Methods of assessment should depend upon what is being assessed. If we think back to Scenario 7.1, when Yasmeen undertakes an aseptic wound dressing as part of her assessed proficiencies, her assessor could supplement the evidence she has from the direct observation of her performing the skill with some questions afterwards, and feedback from the patient. **Validity** refers to the quality of the assessment; whether it actually measures what it intends to measure. If Yasmeen is required to be able to *demonstrate an aseptic technique,* using questions alone would not be a valid assessment for this. Using more than one method of assessment will increase the validity. The concept of **triangulation** of assessment in educational terms describes how an assessor can use several sources of data or evidence to help make an assessment decision. By using different sources of data, the assessor can verify and compare the data to help them form a more rounded picture of the student's abilities. Applying this to Scenario 7.1, Yasmeen's practice assessor could use a combination of observation, questioning and testimony evidence to help her reach a decision about Yasmeen's proficiencies. **Reliability** of assessments refers to the measure of providing similar results if used on multiple occasions and by different assessors. If an assessment provides an accurate measurement of a student's performance, there should be consistency in results. In the Scenario, the practice assessor uses guidelines that the Trust has developed relating to aseptic techniques. Yasmeen will have been made aware of these guidelines early in the placement by Jan and that these would be used to assess her practice. Using guidelines or criteria for assessing practice aids reliability as it objectifies the skill being assessed and removes any variance that individual assessors could have.

Involving others in assessment decisions

The patient, service user or carer voice has become a principal concept in the quality assurance processes of standards for practice, education and training. There is a requirement that programme providers make it explicit how patients, service users and carers contribute to the assessment process (NMC, 2018b). This recognises and places value on the expertise that patients, service users and carers bring. It is common for practice assessment documentation to include patient/service user/carer feedback forms. This approach is supported by the *Report of the Mid-Staffordshire NHS Foundation Trust Public Inquiry* (Francis, 2013), which recommended a common culture of putting the patient first. In addition, the *Review into the Quality of Care and Treatment Provided by 14 Hospital Trusts in England* identified the need to listen to the views of patients and engage them in service improvement initiatives (Keogh, 2013). Research also highlights the value of feedback from patients, clients, carers and service users which can help with practice assessment decisions (Helminen et al., 2014). Activity 7.3 will help you consider how to best obtain this type of feedback and how to minimise any potential issues with requesting patient feedback and testimonies.

Activity 7.3   Reflection

Think of a time when you have been involved in the assessment of a student in your work area.

- Did you/colleagues use feedback from patients, service users or carers to inform the assessment decision? If so, how was this obtained?
- Thinking about the considerations involved in asking those in care situations for feedback, how could this be improved in your work area?

There is a model answer for this activity at the end of this chapter.

Activity 7.3 highlights that there are many considerations when asking those in vulnerable care situations for feedback. These considerations include: individuals potentially feeling pressured to give feedback; required to be positive; responsible for passing or failing a student; not able to have anonymity; too ill to offer opinion; or that any input might affect their future care (Atkinson and Williams, 2011). Patient, service user and carer input into the student assessment process is, however, fundamental and these considerations can be successfully managed by the practice assessor. Obtaining written feedback and testimonies relating to the student's approach to care, communication, compassion and dignity is invaluable to a robust assessment. If you have an opportunity to develop or revise any documentation, work with relevant stakeholders, for example patients, service users or carers, to ensure the wording and design are appropriate. Remember that consent must be obtained by the registrant, not by the student, for any assessment feedback.

The NMC (2018c) states that practice supervisors would not be expected to carry out summative practice assessments or sign off student proficiency; however, they would contribute to the assessment of students by providing feedback to the practice assessor. This will be strengthened by documenting formative commentary on the student's progress in appropriate learning records such as practice assessment documentation. Feedback from practice supervisors is therefore fundamental to student assessment decisions. Practice supervisors should regularly feed back and update on progress as well as provide testimony evidence towards formal assessments.

Feedback

Receiving feedback is a fundamental part of the learning process. Effective and timely feedback is essential for the student–practice supervisor/assessor relationship in order for the student to learn from their experiences. Feedback has been defined as a process whereby students obtain information about their work in order to appreciate the similarities and differences between the appropriate standards for any given work and the qualities of the work itself, in order to generate improved work (Boud and Molloy, 2013). A literature review examining published research in this area found that feedback was often viewed as challenging to deliver and varied greatly in quality (Pollock et al., 2015). It can be particularly difficult if you are required to feed back on an area of the student's practice that needs improving, and not surprisingly, many individuals involved in supporting practice learning reported that they found it much easier to provide positive feedback. Activity 7.4 is designed to help you enhance your feedback skills.

Activity 7.4   Reflection

Think back to a time when you gave some feedback to a student. You might have been giving positive feedback or giving feedback to a student who was struggling or failing to achieve.

- How did you do this?
- How was it received?
- How did you determine that the student understood the feedback?
- Would you do anything differently next time?

If you have not yet had any experience of giving feedback to a student, think of a time you have provided feedback to another individual.

There is no model answer for this activity as it refers to your own experience, but there are some related key points about feedback provided at the end of this chapter.

Activity 7.4 helps you to think about how feedback is received and reminds us that feedback is a two-way process. You will be able to learn and develop from the feedback provided by the students you are working with in relation to your supervisory or assessor skills. All feedback should be constructive, i.e. to help the individual progress and improve. Constructive feedback does not mean only giving positive feedback or praise. It also means giving negative feedback skilfully so that it is useful. Destructive feedback is unhelpful and describes negative feedback given in an unskilled way that leaves the student feeling bad with nothing to build upon. Constructive feedback must be specific and different to general everyday comments you might use like *that's fine* or *keep practising*, etc. Constructive feedback should include detail on performance in reference to relevant criteria, so the student is clear about their progression.

There are recognised principles and characteristics of good and constructive feedback (Duffy, 2013; Boud, 2015; Scott, 2014). An awareness of these can help us develop our feedback style and skills. Good and constructive feedback is:

- specific, focused on behaviour that can be changed, not on perceived attitudes or generalisations;
- accurate, factual and based on observation;

- objective, unbiased and unprejudiced;
- timely, given in good time, as soon as possible after the *event*;
- constructive, about what the individual did well and what they could do better, related to goals so the student is able to *use* the feedback;
- ready to be received, to aid motivation. Timing and location can help – feedback is best given in private;
- well communicated. Use principles of good communication to deliver the feedback and check for understanding.

It can be helpful when developing our own feedback skills to recognise constructive feedback in other conversations. Scenario 7.2 is an excerpt from a conversation where Jan provides feedback to Yasmeen following a clinical procedure.

Scenario 7.2

Jan has observed Yasmeen undertaking an aseptic wound dressing on an elderly male patient with a leg ulcer. After Yasmeen has finished the procedure, Jan provides her with some feedback. Here is an excerpt from their conversation.

Jan: *How did you feel about undertaking the wound dressing today?*

Yasmeen: *Ok, I guess. I think I did a good job but I'm not sure if I missed anything.*

Jan: *Are you ready for me to provide you with some feedback?*

Yasmeen: *Yes please.*

Jan: *I will work through the criteria related to this clinical procedure and give you feedback on each stage. You clearly obtained verbal informed consent from the patient and I particularly liked how you repeatedly checked his understanding of the procedure before you got started. You followed the Trust procedure for decontaminating your hands both pre and post the procedure and I noted that you took care to remove your watch and wash your wrists. You prepared your sterile field as we have been practising, and because you were familiar with the equipment, this seemed to help you to keep exposure of the wound to a minimum. You followed the care plan and redressed the wound as the plan required. I could see you had a close look at the wound and old dressing, what were you looking for?*

Yasmeen: *I was looking for any signs of wound infection and checking there wasn't any irritation from the old dressing.*

Jan: *Well done! I thought that might be what you were doing. You maintained asepsis throughout. I thought you managed that very well, especially as the patient tried to wriggle his leg at one point, but you were quick to notice and explain why you*

---

needed him to keep still. One criterion that you didn't fully meet was maintaining the patient's comfort and dignity throughout the procedure. Although you started the procedure by ensuring he was comfortable, you didn't seem to notice your patient's body language during the procedure. At one point he looked really uncomfortable. Did you notice this?

Yasmeen: *I think I was too busy focusing on getting the skill right that I forgot to keep checking on his comfort. I will make sure next time that I regularly ask the patient how they are and try and be more observant of their body language.*

Jan: *Yes, that would be good. I appreciate there is a lot to focus on when developing your new skills. Try and keep open communication channels throughout the procedure and you will quickly be aware if your patient is uncomfortable. I think in this instance, explaining that you were removing a dressing and it could feel uncomfortable for a few minutes would have really helped with this. Have I been clear that this one criterion was not fully met, which means you will need to be assessed again against this proficiency?*

Yasmeen: *Yes, I understand.*

Jan: *Ok. To continue, I think your documentation of the procedure is clear and detailed and I was especially impressed with your detailed description of the wound.*

Activity 7.5   Evidence-based practice and research

Using your knowledge of principles and characteristics of constructive feedback, read through Scenario 7.2 and think about the conversation between Jan and Yasmeen.

- Does Jan provide Yasmeen with constructive feedback?
- Find examples from the conversation to support your answer.

There is a model answer at the end of this chapter.

Constructive feedback can: promote improvement and development; sustain and increase motivation; increase confidence and self-esteem; increase competence and improve quality of care; promote open communication channels; and create a feedback-friendly culture across the wider team, which helps teams improve (Boud, 2015). These benefits are fundamental for the student but are also noted as being beneficial for the supervisor or assessor who is providing the feedback. If we consider Jan's feedback to Yasmeen in Scenario 7.2, we can see that she largely covered the principles and characteristics of constructive feedback.

Feedback models

Models can provide a structure to the feedback process and are particularly useful when we are developing and refining our skills as supervisors and assessors. There are a range of feedback models available, and you might find that one particular one works better for your own communication style and your students. Table 7.2 summarises four commonly used models or approaches to feedback in clinical practice.

Feedback model/ approach	Description	Uses
The feedback sandwich	This model consists of three parts where you make positive statements, discuss areas for improvement and then finish with more positive statements.	This aims to minimise the potential for any detrimental effect of discussing the *negative* aspect.
The stop – start – continue	This model consists of three parts where you discuss with your student what they feel they should stop doing; what they feel they should start doing; and what they wish to continue doing.	This aims to give the feedback some structure, ensuring the negative part is addressed, but acknowledging the positives to *carry on.*
The situation – behaviour – impact	This approach consists of three stages where you begin with defining the situation the feedback refers to; next define the specific behaviours you want to address; and end by describing how those behaviours affected you or others.	This allows the student to reflect on their actions while understanding specifically what you are commenting on and why, as well as think about what they need to change.
Pendleton's model of feedback	This model has several stages: 1. Check the student is ready for feedback. 2. The student gives a background to the event/procedure that is being assessed. 3. The student states what was done well. 4. The supervisor/assessor(s) states what was done well. 5. The student states what could be improved. 6. The supervisor/assessor(s) states how it could be improved. 7. An action plan for improvement is made, in partnership between student and supervisor/assessor.	This approach encourages the student to identify areas of improvement, which are then followed by discussion with the supervisor/assessor.

Table 7.2 Commonly used feedback models in clinical practice

You might find that you adapt a model to better fit your individual style. Being aware of which approach or model you use can be helpful in developing your skills as well as checking that you work through the stages fully. Activity 7.6 provides an opportunity to explore your feedback style a little further.

Activity 7.6 Reflection

Revisit the experience or event you identified in Activity 7.3.

- Did you use a model to structure your feedback? If so, which one?
- Do you have a preference towards any of the models outlined in Table 7.2? Now think about how you would have delivered the feedback using the preferred model.

There is no model answer as this activity relates to your experiences. However, components of feedback models are further outlined at the end of this chapter.

You may have noted from undertaking Activity 7.6 that you use different feedback styles or models depending upon the type of feedback you are giving. Feedback can sometimes be difficult to give and receive, especially if your student is underperforming. Remember, constructive feedback should always be given in a way that supports professional development. Creating a feedback culture in your workplace means that you support and encourage all kinds of feedback, for colleagues as well as students. Feedback for positive behaviours and practice often gets neglected and forgotten, and you can start to practise this in your own practice setting. Encouraging all types of feedback results in it ultimately becoming easier when you need to give and receive negative feedback.

Students in difficulty

What happens when our students are failing to meet their objectives during their clinical placement? Students might be struggling and *in difficulty* – and we can help as their practice supervisors or practice assessors. The term *in difficulty* in this context is defined by Health Education England (HEE) (2015) as when a student has "a problem(s) in their education, training, conduct or health that affects, or is likely to affect significantly, patient safety, team working, educational progress or their well-being". It is a term commonly used by health professionals, particularly in medicine and dentistry. It is used to explore students' situations, and also situations registered practitioners might find themselves in at various points of their careers.

We all vary in our capacity for self-regulation of our emotions and this is further compounded by the particular context and physical and psychological state we happen to be in. The emotions involved when a student is struggling could manifest themselves as anger, fear, hostility and disappointment. This might result in a display of difficult behaviours, for example rudeness; hostility; impatience; and avoidance. Findings from research studies show that in this situation, the possibility for further errors increases whilst the individual's overall confidence levels drop. In addition, the interpersonal relationship between the struggling student and others deteriorates, as the frustration between themselves and their supervisors/assessors builds. This is compounded as more people become aware and involved in the situation (Evans and Brown, 2017), for example academics from the student's course. All these factors add to the student's rising stress levels. In Scenario 7.3 we consider some of the signs and behaviours a student in difficulty might display.

Scenario 7.3

This Scenario outlines a conversation between Kate, a practice supervisor, and Jez, a first-year student. Jez is halfway through his first placement, and he has been working most of the previous four weeks with Kate. At the start of the week, Kate discussed with Jez at his midpoint interview how she was concerned with his progression towards his placement outcomes. Today Kate takes Jez to a quiet area before they start their shift together to talk more about this, based on events from the previous day. The conversation outlines some of the behaviours a struggling student might be displaying.

Kate: *Do you feel like you've made any more progress towards your outcomes since we spoke last week?*

Jez: *I thought I was until I totally messed up with Mr Davidovic's personal care yesterday. After that it's all gone downhill, I just can't seem to get anything right.*

Kate: *I know that you didn't help him to get washed and dressed in time for his tests as we had planned, but later that day once I'd helped him, he was happy enough with the care he'd received.*

Jez: *That's good to hear!*

Kate: *I was surprised you weren't around to help me with his care, in fact I didn't see you for the rest of the shift yesterday. What were you doing?*

Jez: *(tearful) I'll never be able to do it like you. I didn't think Mr Davidovic would want me anywhere near him after I messed up with getting him ready on time. I think he'll feel better if I'm not involved in his care anymore.*

Kate: *So you just left him and our other patients?*

Jez: *I thought it better if I went to the day room and looked through those folders you showed me from the office, the ones full of information about treatment procedures.*

Kate: *Really Jez, that wasn't a good time to be reading about treatments; you left me with lots to do! Today I'd like you to work with Mr Davidovic again; you can start by helping him with his personal care.*

Jez: *(looks uncomfortable, sighs and walks towards the patient's room)*

In Scenario 7.3, we can sense the rising frustration for both parties through the developing conversation. Jez's confidence in his ability to undertake care for Mr Davidovic is low. This is causing him to avoid direct caring opportunities. Kate is asking Jez to work with Mr Davidovic again as she thinks this will help him confront his anxieties. However, this seems to have resulted in Jez's stress levels rising as he is now in an *uncomfortable* position and could potentially put the patient's safety and wellbeing at risk.

Recognising students in difficulty

If a student is failing to meet their proficiencies, you might try further simulation of the assessment task with your student. This could involve role play; simulation aids, for example human mannequins; or further demonstration from yourself or colleagues. Coaching approaches can really help here. In Scenario 7.2 Jez might benefit from observing Kate provide more direct care episodes with patients, before being asked to undertake this again on his own. Further exposure to the situation, more time or supported further attempts can really make a difference. Chapter 4 highlights different learning styles that can help us to understand behaviours. Sometimes students have difficulty transitioning learning from the classroom into the clinical environment. Simulation can bridge this type of difficulty, and you can facilitate this by providing a safe environment to *practise* the desired skill or behaviour before undertaking it for real. Chapters 5 and 6 of this book outline different teaching methods to further encourage student engagement.

Professional courses like nursing and midwifery require students to have clinical knowledge, skills and attitudes embedded throughout the course. Students are also required to demonstrate high standards of professional conduct at all times, and these are embedded in assessments. A student in difficulty might be able to meet their placement proficiencies as they have the relevant skills and knowledge, but may be struggling with the less tangible development of a good professional attitude or values. Undesirable attitudes are often the hardest aspect for practice supervisors and practice assessors to address as they are difficult to objectify. The student might seem unmotivated and disinterested, or might be struggling to engage with patients, yourself or the wider team. They might have poor timekeeping, undesirable ways of communicating or an unsuitable dress code. They could appear anxious or fearful, and as if they are not enjoying the placement. In Scenario 7.2, it is unclear whether it is a skill, knowledge or attitude deficit Jez has or whether there is some other interpersonal difficulty. There are many stressors involved in being a student, and indeed as a registrant. Stress is a part of everyday life and can be very useful. However, some ways in which we respond to stress can be unhelpful and when experienced over a prolonged period, stress can cause us to have physical and psychological problems. NHS Choices (2017) describes stress as "the feeling of being under too much mental or emotional pressure". When we are no longer able to cope with the pressures we are faced with, this turns into stress, which then impacts how we are able to think, act and cope.

Your student might be experiencing problems in their personal life, which is affecting their performance at work. This could include loneliness, relationship problems, financial difficulties and problems with mental or physical health. Being in a stressed state is not always recognisable by the person experiencing it, therefore it is essential for us to recognise potential stress signs in ourselves, students and colleagues around us. Chapter 8 provides further consideration of stress and an overview of common stress signs, symptoms and behaviours.

Imposter syndrome

There is evidence to suggest that some personality characteristics can increase an individual's risk of becoming distressed and in difficulty during placement (Sonnak and Towell, 2001). One of these is imposter syndrome (IS), which is a behaviour characterised by intense feelings of fraudulence when achieving success. This characteristic is commonly linked to registrants and student registrants. IS describes a psychological pattern where an individual has a fear of being exposed as a fraud as they have internal doubts about their achievements. It often manifests itself as feelings of self-doubt, fear that an individual's true abilities will be found out and that other people have an over-inflated perception of that individual's abilities (Jarrett, 2010). Students who experience IS believe they have somehow 'fooled' people into believing they are more intelligent and competent than they really are and believe they don't deserve success; instead they have somehow been lucky *to get away with it* up to this point. A large-scale research study by Christensen et al. (2016) examining IS in nursing students worldwide found younger students and those who had less support in their home life exhibited a higher proportion of imposter-type feelings. They also found that IS manifests itself in times of increased accountability and responsibility, for example during placement assessment periods.

You might recognise IS in your student if they repeatedly express feelings of self-doubt by saying *I'm not as good as you think I am* or have difficulty taking credit for what they have achieved by saying *I don't deserve to pass this*. They might be frustrated and feel unable to meet their self-set standards if they are a perfectionist and unable to accept anything other than the very high level of performance they have set for themselves. An IS personality trait often leads a student to lack in confidence and have an exaggerated fear of making mistakes. In Scenario 7.2, Jez could be experiencing these feelings as he states *I didn't think he'd want me anywhere near him so I kept away. I'll never be able to do it like you. I think he'll feel better if I'm not involved in his care.*

We can support students to overcome fears of under-confidence and IS through effective assessment and feedback. Research studies have found this occurs when students are supported to fail and face disappointment, but in a constructive and supportive way. For example, we could provide practice for tasks (formative), providing multiple opportunities to fail without it being in a high-risk situation (summative). This develops the student's ability to learn from the failing experience in a supportive manner. An example of this could be learning to better receive feedback or learning to reflect on one's own practice. Another suggestion is to discourage students in comparing their own performance to that of others. Instead, they should be comparing their performance to examples of their own earlier performances. If we apply these suggestions to Scenario 7.2, Kate could provide Jez with additional opportunities for direct patient care, providing feedback each time. Kate could also ask Jez to think about other care episodes he has been part of and recognise any development from these. Most importantly, students with IS need to be reminded that they are still developing in their careers, which makes it difficult to actually be an *imposter* (Chapman, 2017).

Supporting the student in difficulty

The aim of support is to move the student out of the *difficulty* that, if it persists, is likely to lead the student to fail. Supportive supervision can really help. This involves: effective communication, a trusting relationship, constructive feedback and choices of learning and assessment methods. Changing or modifying attitudes requires an individual to work on often deep-rooted subconscious beliefs and values, so it requires a lot of effort. Motivation for change must come from the individual student themselves.

There are many models that can be used in a *helping* relationship. One that is particularly useful for students in difficulty is Egan's Skilled Helper model. Traditional approaches to mentoring, coaching and supervision position the *helper* as the expert who identifies what the *problem* is and any subsequent solutions. The student then receives instruction about what to do, with the underpinning philosophy being that knowledge will lead to a change in behaviour. However, this puts the student in a passive position, and rarely results in changed behaviour. Research relating to helping students out of difficulty supports the use of an individual-centred model such as Egan's (Newnham-Kanas et al., 2010). This approach acknowledges the reasons for *struggling* or being *in difficulty* are often complex and multi-faceted. It also acknowledges that the student needs to be driving any changes required. Egan's model positions the student as the expert who, if supported, can identify their own issues and goals. The supervisor or assessor facilitates the process, providing cues for action and reinforcing positive behaviour. This, in turn, results in the student developing skills of self-management as well as resilience. Even when a student is not in difficulty, you might find using elements of this model useful to motivate engagement.

Using Egan's Skilled Helper model with a student in difficulty

Egan's Skilled Helper model is also used in Chapter 8, but it is particularly useful here for students in difficulty as it is concise, offers a staged approach and provides structure and guidance for those in supporting roles. It is recognised as being particularly helpful where there is a goal of long-lasting change required. The model has three stages, which can be summarised as: what is going on; what does the individual want instead; and how can the individual achieve what they want (Egan, 2013)? Let's consider how we can apply the three stages of Egan's model to the characters in Scenario 7.4.

Scenario 7.4

Kate is familiar with Egan's Skilled Helper model and has used this before. Prior to arranging a meeting with Jez, Kate reflects upon how she has used this model previously with students. She writes herself a plan of how she might use the model with Jez, and notes down prompts for her to use at each stage. She plans for Jez to be doing most of the talking in the meeting, and she finds it helpful to make some notes to remind her how to ask open-ended questions. Kate's preparation notes are as follows.

First actions – Arrange a first meeting with Jez, check our schedules and ensure we can have 1 hour uninterrupted. Arrange a suitable room, let Jez know these details.

During the meeting – Work through Egan's three-stage model (although we might need a series of meetings for this).

Stage 1: Telling the story

Aim of the stage – To provide a safe place for the student to tell their story and uncover the current scenario.

Notes – Involves creating a space to hear and understand Jez's story in his own words. I can help him to see the wider picture and any other perspectives, finding a point to be able to move forwards. I should be aiming to provide hope.

1a: The story – Encourage Jez to talk about what's really going on. Use effective active listening skills including open questions, summarising, paraphrasing and reflecting. Useful questions: How did you feel …? What were you thinking when …? and What else is there about that …?

1b: Blind spots – Help Jez to find out what's really going on, uncovering any gaps in his assessment of the situation. Any impact of his behaviour on others, strengths, etc. I should be challenging, helping Jez to recognise any discrepancies, distortions or if he's not fully aware. Useful questions: How might others see this …? Is there any other way of looking at this …? or What about all of this is an issue for you?

1c: Leverage – Focus and move forward. Help move Jez from being stuck to moving forwards and having hope. Help him to choose an area he has energy to work on to start to move forwards that will make a difference and be of benefit to him. Useful questions: What in all this is the most important to you? What is manageable? and What might make the most difference to …?

Stage 2: The preferred picture

Aim of the stage – To help the student find what they want instead.

Notes – Ensure Jez reflects upon what he really wants from this, instead of jumping straight into a solution to what he's identified as an issue in stage 1.

2a: Possibilities – Help Jez to brainstorm his ideal scenario; note down brainstorm ideas. Make sure I am non-judgemental and don't add my solutions – this is Jez's ideal scenario. Encourage blue-sky thinking here and for him not to be shackled with practicalities. Encourage Jez to be creative and imaginative to generate energy. Useful questions: What do you ideally want instead? What would be happening …? and What would you be doing/thinking/feeling?

2b: Change agenda – Help Jez to reflect upon his brainstorm ideas and formulate goals which are SMART (Specific, Measurable, Achievable, Realistic and Time-phased). Useful questions: What exactly is your goal with this? Which of these feels best for you to address? and Which of these feels manageable to address?

2c: Commitment – Test this is the right goal for Jez to work on, and his commitment to it, before he moves into action. Useful questions: How will it be different for you when you do this? What are the benefits for you in doing this? and What are the disadvantages for you in doing this?

Stage 3: Finding a way forward

Aim of stage – To help the student with how to get to where they want.

Notes – Help Jez identify any strategies or actions to be able to move towards his identified goals as well as considering what/who could help or hinder this.

3a: Possible actions – Help Jez to brainstorm strategies to achieve his goal. Again, encourage blue-sky thinking as ideas for action might come from wild ideas. Useful questions: What are the ways in which you could achieve …? Who/what could help? and What has helped/hindered before?

3b: Best fit strategies – Help Jez to focus from the brainstorm ideas on what is realistic for him and best fits with his circumstances and values. Useful questions: Which of these ideas appeals to you most? Which of these ideas is most likely to work? and Which of these ideas do you have the resources to do?

3c: Plan – Help Jez to plan the next steps by breaking down the goal into smaller steps for action. I must ensure this is Jez's plan and timescales, and not my own. Useful questions: What will you do first of all? When will you achieve this by? and What will you need to do next?

End actions – Jez should have an action plan and begin to start working to this, whilst we still have regular meetings regarding the plan's progress. The plan/goal may need revising or adjusting.

Activity 7.7   Critical thinking

Read through Scenario 7.4 – Kate's preparation notes for meeting with Jez.

1. What sort of communication style is Kate planning to use? How do we know this?
2. Think about your own communication style and skills. What are your strengths and weaknesses regarding communication skills? You might find this helpful to note down.

There is a model answer for this activity at the end of this chapter.

Egan's Skilled Helper model is useful to provide us with a framework or map to then be able to explore issues affecting the student, and help them to move to action. The model is designed to keep the student's agenda central, and we can see from Kate's plan in Scenario 7.2 and your critical thinking from Activity 7.7 that her role is to prompt and ask open-ended questions of Jez. She aims to enable him to end up with a plan of action for himself, developed from his own goals. Principles of good active listening are required throughout this interaction, and it's important that Kate doesn't try and add her own *solutions* but instead works in a very facilitative way to help Jez through the stages to reach his own. Not every student will need to address all three stages, and at times individuals may move back into previously addressed stages. Kate might find she uses her plan sequentially as she has written it, but she will also have to be prepared to work with Jez in all or any of the stages, and move backwards and forwards, as needed. It is not uncommon for the student to revisit earlier stages as the issue they first identified isn't the one they most want to address. Not all the stages will take an equal amount of time to work through, and this will vary depending on the student and also on their particular *issue*. Kate might find that it takes up all of one or maybe more meetings for Jez to work through stage 1, yet the following stages might then happen relatively quickly as the student begins to pick up pace as they move to action. The key with using this model is flexibility.

Supporting the failing student

Most students will achieve their required proficiencies in practice. Indeed, most students *in difficulty* who are provided with support will go on to achieve and pass the placement. However, there are a few students whose performance is not able to meet the required standards even with extra support, and these students will need to be supported to fail practice. It is not always straightforward to be able to fail a student. *Failure to fail* is the term used when students who do not display satisfactory clinical performance are given a pass mark. Duffy's (2003) seminal work on failing to fail showed that mentors were sometimes passing students they thought should have failed. The reasons for this were that mentors lacked confidence in failing students and wanted to give students the *benefit of the doubt*. Failing to fail can have significant implications for the students and practice assessors involved, as well as an effect on nursing professionalism and in particular patient safety. Duffy's work led to a revision in the NMC (2008) guidance for those supporting practice assessments. However, more recent research has shown that failing to fail still occurs. Registrants involved in assessment decisions often struggle to deal with personality clashes, emotional blackmail, poor hygiene, aggression, punctuality and learning difficulties such as dyslexia (Lawson, 2010). Activity 7.8 offers you an opportunity to explore these issues further.

Activity 7.8   Leadership and management

Using any experiences you may have had in working with failing students, think about potential reasons why failing to fail still happens.

If you haven't had any direct experiences of working with failing students, you could ask your colleagues about their experiences. You might find it helpful to make a note of these.

There is a model answer at the end of this chapter that outlines common themes about failing to fail from the wider literature.

Assessment of competence is an essential component of the practice assessor's role. Activity 7.8 highlights that failing a student can be difficult for many reasons, and sometimes results in failing to fail.

Indicators of failing practice

Earlier in this chapter, indicators of students being in difficulty were highlighted. However, there are also common indicators in a student's skills performance or behaviour, which could alert an assessor to the possibility of failure. Table 7.3 outlines common indicators of student practice failure from research undertaken by Duffy and Hardicre (2007a). You might recognise some of the indicators from students you have already worked with and reflections from Activity 7.8.

Utilising the assessment process

One of the factors Duffy (2003) found that contributed to registrants failing to fail was that those undertaking practice assessments lacked knowledge of the assessment process. It should be very clear for the student whether the assessment is formative

Common indicators of student practice failure

- Inconsistency in meeting the required level of competence for the stage of training;
- Inconsistent clinical performance;
- Lack of insight into weaknesses so unable to change following constructive feedback;
- Unsafe practice;
- Not responding appropriately to feedback;
- Lack of interest or motivation;
- Limited practical, interpersonal and communication skills;
- Absence of professional boundaries and/or poor professional behaviour;
- Experiencing continual poor health, feeling depressed, uncommitted, withdrawn, sad, tired or listless;
- Unreliability, persistent lateness/absence;
- Preoccupation with personal issues;
- Lack of theoretical knowledge.

Table 7.3 Common indicators of student practice failure (Duffy and Hardicre, 2007b)

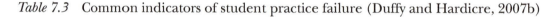

or summative. Students should usually have at least three formal meetings with their practice assessor. There should be an initial assessment interview, mid-placement interview and final placement interview. These are particularly helpful for highlighting progression and any issues.

At the initial meeting, it is essential to discuss any learning needs and requirements. The student's documentation should be reviewed and then, between assessor and student, any learning objectives and action plans should be developed. Future meetings should be scheduled, and all this activity thoroughly documented.

The mid-placement interview is formative and it is crucial to highlight the student's progress towards their objectives and plans at this point. Any areas for development should be discussed here, especially if the practice assessor has any concerns about the student's progression. Any conversations of this nature along with any plans for development, records of extra support required and other actions should be thoroughly documented. If there are concerns regarding progression at this point, it will also be necessary to contact the student's academic tutors, who can provide additional support for the student as well as for the assessor. This could be their academic tutor or tutor who links from the AEI, and their contact details should be clearly outlined in the student's assessment book. This meeting is potentially the most critical in supporting failing students because of its timing. It should provide an opportunity for any concerns to be addressed with the student, and support to be put in place to scaffold the rest of the placement. With additional support and action plans, the aim is for the student to be able to successfully progress and achieve their outcomes. Assessors should not leave the failing news to the last meeting where there is no chance of the student being able to correct the situation. Duffy (2003) found that mentors often failed to fail because of a fear that their decision would be *overruled* by the student's AEI. Students are only able to appeal a failed assessment decision if there are grounds on which to do so. If the assessor fails to highlight concerns at this midpoint, it would be a case for appeal as the student has not had time to address any weaknesses or flaws.

The final assessment interview will include summative assessment decisions and should take place towards the end of the placement. There should be no surprises for the student at this meeting, as concerns and progress have been discussed previously. The meeting is used to record a pass or fail grade for the placement. Each AEI will have its own set of documentation to use for these meetings and it is critical for the practice assessor to familiarise themselves with the documentation used in their area. It is also important for practice supervisors to be familiar with assessment documentation and how the student is progressing. Supervisors will be responsible for feeding into assessment decisions and will need to be cognisant of any objectives, action plans and additional support that have been planned. Failing a student can be a difficult and unpleasant experience for the practice assessor, as well as the wider team involved in supporting the student. The important factor throughout this assessment process is that you seek support as early as possible for yourself as well as your student, if there are causes of concern regarding progression.

Student reactions to failing decisions

Upon hearing that they are underperforming or failing a placement, students can act in numerous ways. As with any bad news, it will take time to digest what is being said and you might find you need to repeat information given, or even write down information for the student. Table 7.4 outlines numerous student reactions to failing decisions. You might be familiar with these reactions if you have been involved in breaking bad news to patients or service users. It is likely you will already have transferable communication skills with delivering the bad news, in this instance to students instead of patients/service users.

Potential student reactions	Explanations for reactions
Denial, disbelief and shock	The student may have an inaccurate self-assessment of their own abilities and competence. Alternatively, they might have received differing feedback from other colleagues who gave them the *benefit of the doubt*.
Betrayal	The student might feel hurt that their practice assessor and/or supervisor, who they felt they got along well with, could fail them.
Sadness and upset	The student might cry or be tearful.
Anger, aggression and denial	The student may shout or verbally abuse their practice assessor, accusing them of bias or victimisation.

(Continued)

Table 7.4 (Continued)

Potential student reactions	Explanations for reactions
Blaming others	The student might blame personality clashes or accuse the assessor of underperforming themselves. The student may blame others for giving them the wrong information. This could be the assessor, previous assessors, other members of the team, academics or even other students.
Bargaining, coercion	Some student nurses can use coercive and manipulative behaviour to try and gain a successful outcome to their practice learning assessment. They might try and bargain with the assessor to change their assessment decision. This often results in causing assessors to feel guilty.
Relief	Some students may be relieved and accept a failed assessment. This might be when they themselves have recognised some clinical weakness or areas that need additional work.

Table 7.4 Student reactions to failing decisions (adapted from Duffy and Hardicre, 2007a; Hunt et al., 2016)

An awareness of potential reactions to failing news can really help us prepare for those difficult conversations. These potential reactions also highlight the importance of ensuring you and the student are supported with this process. An academic from the student's programme will ideally be present when news of failing is first presented to the student and then at each meeting where progression is discussed.

Managing failing students

Any concerns about a student's performance should be raised as early as possible. The aim is to provide feedback that can *correct* the concern and support the student to pass. Feedback should be both written and verbal and you may need to arrange several opportunities to keep discussing this so that the student is very clear on what they need to do to improve. Feedback is essential and Chapter 5 outlines principles of good feedback that are particularly helpful here.

Documenting concerns in the student's assessment documentation makes these clear and transparent for the student and all those involved in supporting them. This is especially important if your student is being supervised in practice by a team of supervisors, providing continuity of approach and focus on a shared goal. Evidence should also be documented of related performance and behaviours that are causing the concern. Documenting particular examples can help the student (and others) to better understand assessment decisions. Documentation should be factual; non-judgemental; specific; and identify strengths and weaknesses. All related assessment conversations and details of any supportive measures in place should be recorded.

If issues have been identified, it is important to involve academics from the student's programme and also allocate more supervised time for the student from practice supervisors and assessors. When making an assessment decision, a practice assessor should judge if some minor issues can be accepted as part of the student's continued development, or whether issues are serious and have not been resolved, to the point that failure is inevitable.

Duffy and Hardicre (2007b) offer the following practical tips for dealing with managing failing students:

- Ensure all meetings take place in a private area where you will not be disturbed.
- Invite the student to undertake a self-assessment.
- Formulate an action plan.
- Clearly identify evidence of success or improvements.
- Formulate learning objectives for the next meeting.
- Identify appropriate learning opportunities to meet the objectives.
- Identify additional knowledge required and where the student can access this.
- Plan the date of the next meeting and have regular progress meetings.

Practice assessors and practice supervisors should remain positive and supportive when working with a failing student. Students will have an opportunity to develop over the wider programme even if they have not met the final standard required to pass the particular placement you are assessing. If they have failed the placement, the academic course team will decide on next options for the student. This might be re-taking a particular placement or set of practice assessments or could be moving to an earlier progression point of the course. In some cases, students will be required to leave the course. These decisions are made following a thorough review of the student's profile and any particular assessment patterns. All those involved in supporting assessment decisions should have a sound understanding of the assessment process and be confident in failing a student should they need to. Most importantly, as practice assessors and supervisors, you must be confident that patients and service users will be in safe hands if the student continues to proceed beyond the placement.

Chapter summary

This chapter has introduced you to the key concepts of assessment and feedback. It has provided an overview of assessment methods and quality issues relating to assessment as well as helping us to better recognise and support a student who is in difficulty or failing their summative practice assessment. By completing the activities you will have considered the practice assessment documentation that students bring with them to your practice area and started to familiarise yourself with the students' programmes

(Continued)

(Continued)

and curricula. You will have reflected upon how you use patient/service user or carer feedback as assessment evidence, the benefits of this and potential issues associated with this. You will also have reflected upon your feedback style and the importance of constructive feedback for learning and progression. Through the Scenarios, we noted how proficiencies could be assessed as well as the principles of good feedback. With an increased focus on students working with a range of practice supervisors, we considered how others can effectively support assessment decisions.

Through the chapter Scenarios, we have also considered students in difficulty and how to use a model to support them to achieve. Failing a student's practice assessment is hard and often evokes challenging responses from students. Utilising the assessment process to manage failing students can provide us with a framework to ensure our decisions are fair, transparent and based on evidence. We must be confident that the assessment decisions we are involved with have patient and service user safety at their core.

Activity answers

Activity 7.1: Critical thinking (p132)

There is no correct answer to this activity, as it depends on your practice area and the approach of the AEIs you work with. However, you have probably noticed that the focus is on tasks and direct observation that are consistent with the behaviouristic approach. Although this approach has its critics, it is useful, especially in professions such as nursing and midwifery, which have many tasks and observable behaviours. This is because individual tasks are easily visible, so the assessment document can be used by multiple assessors while the student moves through the programme to different placements.

Activity 7.3: Reflection (p140)

There is no correct answer to this activity, as it depends on your experience and practice setting. However, you may have already developed, or may consider developing, a template to use to obtain student feedback or testimonies. Feedback could be in the form of a short questionnaire or set of cue questions. You might include a scale for individuals to *rate* a professional behaviour if this is to be assessed. Templates for testimonies could include prompts for areas you would like feedback on. Information about using the templates would be useful, reminding individuals of what this is for, how it will be used, what is required and rights to anonymity or to be able to refuse to undertake this without any impact upon their care.

Activity 7.4: Reflection (p141)

There is no correct answer to this activity as it relates to your experiences; however, you might find it useful to read the article by David Boud (2015): Feedback: ensuring that it leads to enhanced learning. *The Clinical Teacher*, *12*(1): 3–7. He summarises with the following key points about feedback:

- Learning involves bridging the gap between desired and actual performance.
- Feedback comments must primarily be judged on their effects on learning and performance.

- It is necessary to look beyond the immediate task: acts of assessment must be designed to leave students better equipped to learn further.

- Learners need to develop a view about what constitutes quality work if they are to demonstrate it for themselves.

- Feedback is not a unilateral act by tutors or trainers, but is a set of interlinked activities.

- Students need always to be positioned by tutors and other staff as proactive learners who can initiate feedback-seeking behaviour.

- Knowledge of the desires and expectations of the student is needed for effective input.

- Effective learning requires dialogue.

- The overriding purpose of feedback is the refinement of the student's capacity to use information to judge themselves in similar situations.

- Inputs from tutors are important as they can open up or close down learning possibilities.

Activity 7.5: Evidence-based practice and research (p143)

Yes, Jan does provide Yasmeen with constructive feedback.

The table highlights some of the evidence you might have noted from Scenario 6.2.

Principles and characteristics of good feedback	Evidence from Jan's feedback to Yasmeen
Specific	Jan provides specific and detailed feedback about a particular care episode.
Accurate	Jan has observed the care episode and asks questions to Yasmeen during the feedback to clarify any area she is unsure of.
Objective	Jan uses the criteria from Yasmeen's skills documentation and Trust's guidelines to structure the feedback, and judge performance.
Timely	Jan provides feedback in a timely way, soon after the care episode and away from the patient/carer or any colleagues.
Constructive	Feedback is specific and focuses on the care episode; where criteria not met, suggestions for ways to develop practice are offered.
Ready to be received	Jan checks that Yasmeen is ready to receive feedback about this event.
Well communicated	Jan uses appropriate questioning, clear language related to the event and checks for understanding.

Activity 7.6: Reflection (p145)

There is no correct answer to this activity as it relates to your experiences; however, whichever model you choose to use, or indeed adapt to work best for you, there are four general components to any model or approach you take. Four general characteristics for feedback models are suggested by Askew and Lodge (2000) and these summarise nicely the components of any good feedback:

1. Involve students in conversation about learning which raises their awareness of quality performance.

2. Facilitate feedback processes through which students are encouraged and motivated to monitor and evaluate their own learning.

3. Enhance student capacities for lifelong learning by supporting their development of skills for goal setting and action planning for learning.

4. Design (formative) assessment tasks in which feedback from varied sources is encouraged, generated, processed and used to enhance their performance.

Activity 7.7: Critical thinking (p152)

1. You will have noticed that Kate plans to use active listening skills in this meeting. This means she will make a conscious effort to hear the words that Jez is saying along with the complete message he is communicating. This involves using open-ended questions, reflection and summarising skills to be absolutely clear of the student's message.

2. There is no model answer for this question as it involves your own experience. However, studies have found that many health professionals don't routinely use active listening skills (Arnold and Boggs, 2015). Instead, we are used to employing a series of closed-ended questions and making quick judgements to then offer our advice. Good communication skills require a high level of self-awareness, so understanding our own style and any development needs is important. If you would like to read further about active listening skills, check out the online resource provided by NHS Improvement (2018) at https://improvement.nhs.uk/documents/2085/active-listening.pdf.

Activity 7.8: Leadership and management (p153)

There is no correct answer to this activity as it relates to your own experiences. However, Hughes et al. (2016) undertook a systematic integrative literature review to determine what is currently known about the issue of *failure to fail* in undergraduate nursing and midwifery programmes. From this research, five main themes emerged concerning why failing to fail still happens. Your list may contain similar issues to those noted by the researchers. These themes were:

1. Failing a student is difficult to do.

2. Failing a student is an emotional experience for all parties involved.

3. Confidence and skills to fail are required to fail students.

4. AEI support is required to fail students.

5. Some student characteristics make failing even more difficult.

The researchers concluded that failure to fail is still a real issue that has many complex facets.

Further reading

Pollock, CHF, Rice, AM and McMillan, A (2015) *Mentors' and Students' Perspectives on Feedback in Practice Assessment: A Literature Review.* NHS Education for Scotland.

This review provides some interesting insights into feedback and its role in practice assessment. The findings section explores how we can seek and use feedback from others in helping support assessment decisions.

Hughes, LJ, Mitchell, M and Johnston, AN (2016) 'Failure to fail' in nursing: a catch phrase or a real issue? A systematic integrative literature review. *Nurse Education in Practice, 20*: 54–63.

This article details the issues involved in failing a student and the emotional processes involved for both assessors and students. It also highlights the implications of failure to fail for the profession, organisations and patient safety.

Chapter 8

Developing yourself as a supervisor and/or assessor

Standards Framework for Nursing and Midwifery Education (NMC, 2018d)

This chapter will address the standard: **3: Student empowerment**.

3.2 Students are empowered and supported to become resilient, caring, reflective and lifelong learners who are capable of working in interprofessional and interagency teams.

It will also address: **4: Educators and assessors**.

4.1 Theory and practice learning and assessment are facilitated effectively and objectively by appropriately qualified and experienced professionals with necessary expertise for their educational roles.

The Code: Professional Standards of Practice and Behaviour for Nurses and Midwives (NMC, 2015)

This chapter most closely aligns with the following professional standards.

Practise effectively

6.2 maintain the knowledge and skills you need for safe and effective practice.

8.4 work with colleagues to evaluate the quality of your work and that of the team.

9.1 provide honest, accurate and constructive feedback to colleagues.

9.4 support students' and colleagues' learning to help them develop their professional competence and confidence.

Preserve safety

16.6 protect anyone you have management responsibility for from any harm, detriment, victimisation or unwarranted treatment after a concern is raised.

(Continued)

(Continued)

Promote professionalism and trust

20.8 act as a role model of professional behaviour for students and newly qualified nurses and midwives to aspire to.

22.3 keep your knowledge and skills up to date, taking part in appropriate and regular learning and professional development activities that aim to maintain and develop your competence and improve your performance.

Chapter aims

After reading this chapter, you will be able to:

- define and describe mental wellbeing and resilience and understand their value within the context of healthcare and supporting learners;
- describe models and techniques to develop resilience and mental wellbeing;
- consider your role as an evidence-informed practitioner;
- assess and plan for your continuing professional development needs;
- apply your knowledge and skills to develop your colleagues and profession.

Introduction

The evidence indicates that being resilient is a protective factor for healthcare professionals (Dean, 2012). Much has been written about the value of resilience in promoting mental wellbeing and protecting healthcare practitioners from burnout and ill-health (Koen et al., 2011). Resilience and mental wellbeing can have a positive effect on absenteeism and is therefore of importance to the NHS, where costs due to ill-health totalled £1 billion in the three-year period preceding 2013 (Anonymous, 2013). Although much has been written about stress and resilience in healthcare, little is known about the impact of resilience in the context of supporting learners, so this chapter will focus on what we do know. It will also consider how resilience can protect patients from harm, through enabling professionals to stay well; can support students who escalate concerns; and can help registrants to fail students who do not meet the required proficiency. The chapter will then move on to look at your how your skills as a practice supervisor/assessor can be used to support your own and your colleagues' professional development, thereby developing your profession as a whole.

What is resilience?

The importance of resilience when experiencing significant life events, such as war and disasters, has been understood for some time. However, resilience has more recently been studied in areas more typical of our daily lives, including working in healthcare. There is evidence to indicate that being a resilient healthcare practitioner not only supports our physical and emotional wellbeing but also offers a level of *protection* in stressful situations, or *when things go wrong* (Seymour-Walsh, 2016).

What do we mean by resilience? The literature suggests that resilient individuals, even after experiencing an adverse event, can function at their previous levels. In addition to maintaining normal functioning, some individuals may also experience increases in autonomy and changes in their perspective on life. In other words, these individuals can change adversity into a positive life experience and *bounce back* stronger than before. Although there are many definitions of resilience, there are a number of shared features:

- the ability to 'bounce back' from a difficult event or experience;
- the ability to hold on to hope and optimism;
- the belief that individuals have a level of influence or control over a situation;
- self-compassion and not blaming oneself;
- the knowledge that resilience is protective.

Resilience can help healthcare practitioners cope with the stresses of the constant decision-making and risk management that they face. Although it is important that we take responsibility for developing our resilience, it is also vital to note that the NHS, as an employer, has a duty to support its staff – especially given they have "very difficult jobs in challenging situations" (Mitchell, 2019). As a result of the COVID-19 pandemic, this level of difficulty and challenge has amplified significantly. A supportive culture at work can have a huge impact on an individual's resilience and ultimately their decision to stay or leave the profession. In addition, staff turnover is costly. Health Education England found turnover costs, linked to a nurse leaving the NHS, range from 0.75 to 2.0 times their salary. Stress is a key factor in nurses' decisions to leave the profession. A recent European study found a staggering 42 per cent of nurses reported burnout, the highest number in Europe (Health Education England, 2014). There are five stages of burnout, and promoting mental wellbeing and resilience may have an impact on preventing movement along the continuum. Therefore, although resilience protects our mental wellbeing and job satisfaction and retention, it is important to reiterate that it is a joint venture; a collaboration between individual and employer. Given its influence on wellbeing and job satisfaction, promoting resilience is a powerful tool to have in both your practitioner and practice supervisor/assessor toolbox. Increasing our self-awareness about our resilience helps us to identify areas that we may find particularly difficult. Activity 8.1 will help with this.

Activity 8.1   Reflection

Resilience checklist

In the table list what boosts your resilience and what erodes it.

Helps	Erodes
e.g. The support I get from my work colleagues	*e.g. Working without a regular lunch break*

There is no model answer as this activity is based upon your own reflection.

Now that you have completed Activity 8.1, think about someone you believe to be resilient. This may be someone you have worked with, or someone you know who has dealt with a difficult situation or life event. Think about their characteristics and attributes and how these link to them being a resilient individual. Now go back to the earlier section which described the features of resilience and identify any *gaps* you have and consider how you might go about acquiring these skills. You may have a coach, supervisor or someone you trust with whom you could talk this over. Consider this as part of your resilience journey and invest in it as it will help protect you for the rest of your career.

Scenario 8.1

This Scenario outlines a day in the life of Tina, an experienced community mental health nurse and practice supervisor, who is working with Daphne, a third-year student nurse.

Tina and Daphne are chatting on the way to a visit. Daphne tells Tina that she is struggling with working in the community and finds it difficult not having a range of colleagues immediately accessible to her. Also, she misses the familiarity of the ward environment, and the sense of 'control' she has there.

Today, they had an appointment with John. John has been diagnosed with paranoid schizophrenia and is very suspicious of Daphne and wonders if she is really a spy. Tina herself is also finding the situation with John hard. She has known him a long time and finds it difficult when he is struggling. However, Tina feels she is able to keep on top of her emotions. Daphne fed back to her that she sees Tina as a positive role model as she remains very caring and compassionate with John while explaining how potentially serious the situation is. Daphne told Tina she hoped she could be as kind and truthful in similar situations.

When they get back to the office, Tina and Daphne hand over to their colleagues and Tina discloses how sad she feels about John's situation and that he may have to be admitted to the hospital: something he really hates.

Later that day, Tina tells Daphne that she is looking forward to a long swim after work because it helps her relax. Also, she has clinical supervision booked in for tomorrow, and this is something she prioritises. The situation with John will be top of her list to discuss. Next week she has a meeting of a journal club she is a member of to discuss developments in her professional field. She enjoys this time learning with and supporting her colleagues. Tina asks Daphne what she plans to do to unwind. Daphne doesn't know.

As highlighted in Scenario 8.1, care and compassion are seen as important aspects of resilience. The 6Cs were launched in 2012 as part of the document *Compassion in Practice* (Cummings and Bennett, 2012) and encompassed the following attributes: care, compassion, courage, commitment, communication and competence. Although the key driver was about adopting and conveying these attributes with patients and carers, they are highly transferable to supporting learners in practice. The summary in Table 8.1 provides an overview of Duffy's (2015) article: Integrating the 6Cs of nursing into mentorship practice.

Complete Activity 8.2 immediately after reading this and consider how adopting the 6Cs in your practice may help you and your learners become more resilient.

Duffy (2015) highlights the importance of role modelling and how both good and bad behaviours and attitudes have a powerful impact on learners.

Care – This can be developed by conveying a sense of belonging to the learners, showing that they are welcome and are part of the team. Encouraging early and active engagement in caring for patients also helps.

Compassion – This can be developed through acknowledging the emotional labour of the work we do and encouraging reflection and including learners in any debriefing following traumatic events. Thinking aloud and sharing your thoughts, including how the situation may be impacting on a patient and their family, demonstrates empathy and compassionate practice to the learner.

Competence – Being supportive in your role as supervisor/assessor enables learners to more readily achieve competence and there are a number of techniques you can use to help develop their psychomotor skills and thereby acquire competence. Supervisor/assessors need to confidently engage learners in a discussion around the evidence base to support their practice and care delivery and the decision around competence.

(Continued)

Table 8.1 (Continued)

> *Communication* – Learners need to be given opportunities to develop their communication skills. Before meeting with a patient, explain to the learner the purpose of the meeting and what you hope to achieve. This will help the learner make sense of the conversation and develop their communication skills. Just as important is role modelling effective communication with members of the wider team, including the university.
>
> *Courage* – Demonstrate to learners you have the passion and courage to innovate and transform practice; to question received wisdom and practices; and to speak out if care isn't good enough. It also takes courage as an assessor to take the decision to fail a learner if they are not achieving the competencies.
>
> *Commitment* – Demonstrate commitment to the supervisor/assessor role and the learner through preparing yourself with the placement documentation, the course and the competencies they need to achieve. This goes beyond the individual and should span the learning environment and the whole team, where everyone is committed to creating a positive learning environment for learners.

Table 8.1 Overview of integrating the 6Cs of nursing into practice learning

As you will have noticed from reading the summary in Table 8.1, role modelling is an important aspect of supporting students.

Activity 8.2   Leadership and management

Identify one change you wish to make against each of the 6Cs in relation to your own practice. You might wish to make a copy of this for your NMC revalidation portfolio and discuss at your appraisal.

There is no model answer for this activity as it is based upon your own reflections.

Acting upon the changes identified in Activity 8.2 will help you to become more resilient. Practice supervisors/assessors who demonstrate the 6Cs also role-model the behaviours of resilient individuals which can help their learners to become more resilient and will help them throughout their career. In Scenario 8.1, Daphne has already noticed that Tina is *very caring and compassionate with John* and is therefore successfully role modelling these behaviours. As a result, Daphne may wish to focus on developing in these areas herself.

Mental wellbeing and resilience

Mental wellbeing contributes to a person being able to develop their potential and work productively and creatively. This enables us to build strong and positive relationships with others and contribute to our community. There are two key aspects of mental wellbeing: feeling good and functioning well. Although it is important to feel happy and engaged, of importance is our sense of purpose in the world and what we can add to it. Many people who choose nursing or midwifery as a career have strong vocational drive to help others and this latter aspect of mental wellbeing may be even stronger. McDermid et al.'s (2016) study of new nurse academics identified three factors that helped them transition into their new role:

- having a mentor and developing supportive work relationships;
- focusing on positive feedback and experiences;
- reflecting on difficult situations and developing as a result of this.

This learning can be applied to students as they transition into new roles. In 2008 the UK government commissioned a mental capital and wellbeing project (Kirkwood et al., 2014). The project identified factors that promote mental wellbeing, termed the *five ways to wellbeing*:

- connect – feeling close to and valued by others;
- be active – enjoying regular physical activity;
- take notice – being mindful and taking time to notice things around you;
- learn – engaging with new learning;
- give – getting involved in community events.

In addition to the five ways to wellbeing, a further resource has been developed by NHS professionals to support employees. Some of this is in relation to working during the COVID-19 pandemic, and the acknowledgement of the toll of this on people's wellbeing. The wellbeing plan is an excellent resource that you could use for yourself and with your learners to help them develop their resilience. It includes an 'emergency reboot' activity, identifying the strategies an individual finds most helpful to them, and a 'people to contact if I feel overwhelmed' exercise (see the further reading section if you would like to try some of these activities).

Activity 8.3   Evidence-based practice and research

1.   Visit Mind's website, which includes more information on the five ways to wellbeing.

(Available online at: **www.mind.org.uk/workplace/mental-health-at-work/ taking-care-of-yourself/five-ways-to-wellbeing**)

2.   Consider each one and identify something you already do or commit to doing something new. Try to ensure you have something against each domain.
3.   Next go back to Scenario 8.1 and identify whether the activities mentioned fit against the five ways.

There is a model answer to the second part of the activity at the end of the chapter.

Developing resilience and mental wellbeing has never been so important. Because of unprecedented working conditions and increased workloads for the entire health and social care workforce as a result of the COVID-19 pandemic, there has been a huge increase in reported levels of burnout and stress. We are all likely to recognise feeling stressed and Table 8.2 outlines some of the common stress signs, symptoms and behaviours (Health and Safety Executive, n.d.).

Emotional	Cognitive symptoms	Behaviours
• Negative or depressive feelings • Disappointment with yourself • Increased emotional reactions – more tearful or aggressive • Loneliness • Loss of motivation, commitment and confidence • Mood swings	• Confusion • Indecision • Inability to concentrate • Poor memory • Lack of clarity • Lack of ability to prioritise	• Changes in eating habits • Increased smoking, drinking or drug-taking activity to cope • Changes in sleep patterns • Twitchy or nervous behaviour • Changes in attendance such as avoidance, arriving later or taking more time off • Withdrawing from others, including social situations

Table 8.2   Common stress signs, symptoms and behaviours

There are many stressors involved in being a student, and indeed as a registered health professional. You might recognise some of the emotional and mental symptoms or changes from normal behaviour outlined in Table 8.2 in yourself and others around you.

Models to help develop your learners' resilience

Activity 8.3 highlighted some basic activities for wellbeing, but there are a number of models that can further develop wellbeing and resilience. Aspects of these models can be used as part of your day-to-day practice when supporting learners. We will now apply Egan's (2013) Skilled Helper model (which is introduced in Chapter 7) and the cognitive behavioural approach. However, regardless of which approach you use, they have the following elements:

- they have boundaries and ground rules – you are the practice supervisor/assessor, not the best friend, nor are you the parent;
- they value the *core conditions*, namely genuineness, warmth and empathy;

- they promote listening and communication skills, including reflecting and paraphrasing;
- they are learner focused – although you have specific tasks to complete, the focus is on the learner's needs. As you know, every learner is different and will have a different set of experiences, strengths, deficits and concerns.

Egan's (2013) Skilled Helper model is discussed here because it is concise and can be applied to supporting learners in practice. Let's consider how we can apply the three stages of Egan's model to the learning environment – where a Learning Environment Manager (LEM) is supporting a new practice supervisor (Table 8.3).

Stage	Attributes, behaviours and activities
Stage 1: telling the story	The LEM spends time with the practice supervisor to understand what they feel are their strengths, concerns and areas for development. The LEM can ask about the situations in which they feel more and less comfortable; the skills they need to develop. Elicit what they have learnt from supporting students. The LEM is mindful not to *take control* of the discussion and to avoid jumping in with answers and advice. *Communication skills such as conveying empathy and compassion will help in this first stage.*
Stage 2: the preferred picture	Once the relationship has been established, the LEM can start to find out what the practice supervisor sees as their goals, such as giving feedback and writing testimonies. *Attributes and skills such as courage and communication will help with this stage.*
Stage 3: finding a way forward	Once both are clear about what needs to be achieved, the LEM can start to create a plan to enable the practice supervisor to get there. They can construct this and adapt it together. The goals should be measurable and achievable. It can be empowering to write a SMART-style goal statement such as 'by July I will have written 10 testimonies and I will feel confident with this activity'. Further information about SMART objectives can be found in Chapter 5. *Skills and attributes such as competence and commitment are important here.*

Table 8.3   Applying the Skilled Helper model

The cognitive behavioural approach suggests that how we react to events is largely determined by our views or beliefs about the event, not the event itself. Therefore, how we think about a situation influences how we feel (emotionally and physically) about it and subsequently how we behave. Through examining and re-evaluating some of our less helpful thoughts and being more self-compassionate, we can develop and try out alternative viewpoints and behaviours that may be more effective in problem-solving and developing resilience (Kemper et al., 2015). The ABC model (adapted from Powell, 2009) helps to further explain this:

A is the **activating event.** This is usually something that happened to the person or something they witnessed or something they are about to experience/take part in

B is their **beliefs**

C is the **consequence(s).** These include how they feel physically, how they feel emotionally and their behaviours – i.e. what they might stop doing, or what they might start to do.

Scenario 8.2 introduces us to David and Ali, and an opportunity to apply the ABC model to the Scenario.

Scenario 8.2

This Scenario focuses on David, a new practice supervisor who is supporting Ali, a second-year nurse. They are working on a busy surgical unit.

Ali and David attended the ward handover, where Ali handed over a patient called Mr Adeboah. Ali forgot to inform the team that Mr Adeboah was nil by mouth in preparation for a procedure to be carried out later. Mr Adeboah was offered a cup of tea later on, which he accepted, and, as a result, his procedure had to be cancelled. The anaesthetist and surgeon complained to the ward manager. David feels very embarrassed that he didn't notice Ali's error and he knows he is accountable. He thinks people are now questioning his competence. He is also worried about the impact this has had on patient care and wonders if this could be considered a near miss. Since this episode, when supervising students David has been constantly double/triple checking that they have passed on all the information, and does not allow them to hand over patient care anymore. This is affecting his students' ability to develop their skills.

Now that you have familiarised yourself with this Scenario, it's time to complete Activity 8.4 and try to apply the ABC model to it.

Activity 8.4   Critical thinking

Read Scenario 8.2 and identify the following:

A: the activating event
B: the beliefs
C: the consequence(s)

There is a model answer at the end of the chapter.

We can see from Scenario 8.2 and Activity 8.4 that what David thinks about the situation (*people will think I am incompetent*) influences how he feels physically and emotionally (*embarrassed*), and then how he behaves (*restricting students' autonomy and double checking everything*). The relationship between these three elements of the ABC model is the key hypothesis in the cognitive behavioural approach (Neenan and Dryden, 2013). This negative spiral may have an impact on David's resilience and ability to *bounce back* as well as role modelling unhelpful behaviours to his students.

However, by disputing negative thoughts (beliefs), we can transform how we think about an event or situation and subsequently what we do (behaviour). The addition of D (dispute) to the ABC model prompts an individual to challenge their negative beliefs, for example considering different thoughts such as: *I should have checked with Ali that he handed that information over, but I didn't as I was so busy it dropped off my list. That doesn't mean I'm incompetent; everyone, even the best supervisors, makes mistakes.*

This may lead to David acting differently, which is the E (or new event) addition to the model. An example of this might be David observing Ali at the next handover for his proficiency in communication. If this new behaviour is repeated on a few separate occasions, and with a range of learners, it should lead to a change in David's behaviour, where he will no longer double/triple check everything, however minor, and a change in his physical and emotional states, where he feels less embarrassed.

Adopting a seven-step, problem-solving sequence (Wasik, 1984, cited in Palmer, 2008) can help practice supervisors or assessors to develop the skills to challenge thinking and change behaviours. The sequence can help guide the conversation and ensure all potential obstacles are taken into account. Table 8.4 applies this sequence to David's situation from Scenario 8.2.

Steps	Questions and actions	David's thoughts and actions
Problem identification	What is the concern?	I've lost confidence in myself as a supervisor.
Goal selection	What do I want?	To feel more confident and allow students some autonomy.
Generation of alternatives	What can I do?	Gradually allow students more autonomy once they have demonstrated competence.
Consideration of consequences	What might happen?	A student might still make a mistake: there's always that risk!
Target	What is the most feasible solution?	Start with patient handover.
Implementation	Now do it!	Starting tomorrow I will gradually allow more autonomy.
		I'll also talk to Ash; he's an experienced supervisor and assessor and someone I trust.
Evaluation	Did it work?	I'll evaluate in one month and get feedback from a range of colleagues, patients and learners.

Table 8.4   A seven-step approach to problem-solving

Dealing with difficult situations

As healthcare professionals, we are constantly dealing with complexity and stressful events. Resilience can help us remain buoyant in the face of these. The COVID-19 pandemic was unprecedented and affected both our professional and personal lives in unimaginable ways. The pace of change in the NHS is fast and constant, and this in itself requires us to be resilient. The NMC has highlighted, in numerous documents, the importance of resilience to the profession and the role it has in enabling registrants to continue to deliver high-quality care. However, we are sometimes faced with very difficult situations or times when things *go wrong*. It is these situations when we need our resilience more than ever in order to bounce back and, if possible, learn from them. In the context of supporting learners, this might be when we make the decision to fail a student or if students we are supporting escalate their concerns about patient safety or sub-standard care.

Duffy (2003) identified the phenomenon of *failing to fail*, which suggested mentors were passing students they thought should have failed. Research carried out by Jervis and Tilki (2011) indicates that this phenomenon is still evident, but they also found that when mentors do make the decision to fail a student, it places intense pressure on them. This is covered in more detail in Chapter 7. Mentors who made the decision to fail a student expressed a range of concerns, including: fear of being subjected to a grievance by the student; worrying that their competence as a mentor might be questioned; having the decision overturned by the university; and feeling emotionally blackmailed by the student. Some experienced stress and sleepless nights. There are a number of recommendations to help practice assessors make the right decisions about a student's progression and how to access support for this. These recommendations include assessor preparation programmes that build in opportunities to reflect on, and critically analyse, experiences in a safe and supportive environment, as well as forums to help practice supervisors and assessors manage difficult situations arising from referring students (Jervis and Tilki, 2011). The benefits of a team approach to supporting learners have been explored in the previous chapters. One of the key drivers of the SSSA was to create distinct roles of supervisor and assessor to promote objectivity and separation between supervision and assessment. This should mean that some of the issues raised by Jervis and Tilki (2011) should be reduced and less emotional toil is placed on assessors.

All learners, whether registrants or students, have a duty to escalate concerns about any poor or dangerous patient care they witness. If students do this during placement, you will need to support them with this. The stress people experience as a result of *whistleblowing* is well documented and a compassionate, supportive response can help the student deal with this (McDonald and Ahern, 2002). Students should be informed at the start of any placement how they can raise concerns and it is recommended they raise any concerns with you initially and also with the AEI. The NMC Code (2015) has many standards relating to raising concerns about public safety. AEIs that deliver pre-registration nurse and midwife education programmes have a protocol readily available to students to assist them to raise concerns. These protocols should be prominent in clinical areas, as this sends a clear message to students that the practice area is open, transparent and takes concerns seriously. It is during these very difficult situations that we need to protect and promote our mental wellbeing, although it is often easy to overlook this. Practising wellbeing techniques when things are going relatively smoothly will set up good habits for when we need to rely on them the most.

The evidence-informed practice supervisor/assessor

Just as your practice as a registered nurse is informed by the evidence base, so should your practice as a practice supervisor/assessor.

This book includes much around the evidence base on coaching, supervising, teaching and assessment, therefore reading this book and completing the activities in it means that you are engaging in evidence-based supervision and assessment. However, what about opportunities to move beyond this and improve your own practice? By this, we mean creating and disseminating evidence and best practice. As a supervisor/assessor of students, you are in a perfect position to do this. This is because almost all of the students you support will be enrolled on an AEI course, be that a nursing degree or something else. Academic colleagues will be supporting you and your colleagues to enable you to best support the students while out on placement. This is your opportunity to engage in collaborations with these staff. Many colleagues at the AEI will be engaged in scholarly activity; this may include undertaking research, postgraduate or doctoral study, presenting at conferences or writing articles and books. Some of this scholarly activity will be focused on practice-based learning and your experience as a practice supervisor/assessor is invaluable and offers you the opportunity to collaborate. For example:

- being a participant in a research project, e.g. your experiences of being a supervisor;
- implementing the recommendations of a research project in your clinical area – such as a new model for supporting students in practice;
- attending as a guest lecturer – to talk about supervising and assessing in practice;
- co-authoring a journal article with a colleague from the AEI – this may be about joint working;
- collaborating on a service improvement project – such as patient involvement in student assessment and feedback.

Assessing and planning for your continuing professional development

Now that you are developing your role as a practice supervisor and/or assessor, the next step is to think about your continuing professional development (CPD) needs in relation to supporting learners.

CPD has a number of definitions but it is the process by which registrants engage in, reflect on and record a range of experiences and learning activities to enhance practice and maintain competence. CPD is a professional requirement for nurses and midwives and the NMC requires all registrants to engage in CPD and return evidence of this as part of the revalidation process (NMC, 2017a). Although there are no legal requirements for employers to support registrants' CPD, many do, as CPD is a critical tool for delivering improved patient health outcomes, ensuring a high-quality health workforce and supporting staff to be safer, more effective and happier (RCN, 2016a). Employers usually support CPD financially and/or through protected study time or you may be eligible for a grant from professional organisations such as the RCN.

CPD can take various forms and includes activities such as formal modules and courses that attract academic credit; conference attendance; working with particular colleagues; or attendance at work-based learning events. Learning can be face to face or online. It also includes keeping up to date with contemporary issues through reading journal articles and books. We may learn with experts in the field including service users, carers and researchers. Many nurses have formal conversations about their CPD needs at their appraisal and as part of the NMC (2017a) revalidation process. You should prepare for these meetings by considering what you believe are your strengths and which areas you would like to develop and then construct an action plan to help you get there – highlighting any support you might need. Consider short-, medium- and long-term goals. Ask at your place of work if there is a buddying or coaching scheme: someone to talk this through with. Professional body websites have invaluable resources and toolkits around career planning and professional development, and you may wish to spend time accessing these.

You may find it useful to review your CPD needs against the *four pillars of advanced practice* (Health Education England, 2017a). These are the four areas that professionals who are working at an advanced level should be competent in: clinical practice; leadership and management; education; and research. What do you need to do to enhance your competence in these areas? You may decide you wish to focus on one area in particular. For instance, you may be interested in a career in nursing or midwifery education either in practice or at an AEI. If that's the case, you could look at job descriptions for such roles and identify the areas you need to develop. Although this may be a longer-term project, you can still begin to develop your skill set and experience now, and Activity 8.5 will help you to explore a CPD opportunity.

Activity 8.5   Evidence-based research

This is your opportunity for some *blue-sky* thinking about your CPD. Imagine you are about to collaborate with a lecturer from your local AEI on scholarly activity in the area of supporting students in practice. What area would you suggest you collaborate on? Look at the list of scholarly activities to help you. Now think about topic areas. What are you particularly interested in? In which areas do you think there are gaps in your knowledge and understanding? What do you think people might like to read or hear about?

Once you have done some free thinking and scribbled down your ideas, start to narrow them down to two or three. Now do the final step, which is to choose one. You might do this rationally and list strengths, limitations and feasibility, etc., or you might go with your *gut feeling*. Now that you have chosen one, why not put together a very brief proposal outlining what the activity is, any background literature and how the scholarly activity might help develop understanding of that area? Ask a colleague who you trust to look at it and then make any amendments you wish to. Now for the hard bit! Contact your AEI link person and ask if you can talk through an idea you have for some scholarly activity.

There is no model answer for this activity as it is based on your own reflections.

Developing and supporting your colleagues and the profession

As a practice supervisor/assessor, in addition to supporting learners you can extend your role to supporting your colleagues' development too. This will help develop the profession, as evidence suggests nurses have a stronger commitment to the profession rather than their employing organisation (Health Education England, 2014). Many of the aspects to your practice supervisor/assessor role highlighted throughout this book can also be applied to supporting colleagues. Some *easy wins* for achieving this are:

- acting as a mentor, coach, preceptor or *buddy* to new or junior staff;
- delivering a learning event to colleagues focused on supporting students;
- co-ordinating activities to support the best use of evidence in practice, such as a journal club;
- facilitating forums or communities of practice for other supervisors/assessors;
- undertaking appraisals with the staff you manage;
- engaging in a reflective discussion (part of the NMC revalidation process);
- acting as a confirmer (part of the NMC revalidation process).

These examples provide an opportunity to support colleagues with their professional and career development goals and for you to provide feedback. These are important because having a good clinical mentor and professional development is likely to improve job satisfaction and retention. However, you can encourage colleagues to step out of their *comfort zones* and consider other activities as part of their CPD. These could include shadowing leaders within the organisation; membership of strategic or clinical excellence groups; presentations at conferences; or getting involved in a service improvement project. The range of CPD opportunities is almost limitless, as you will find when undertaking Activity 8.6. Colleagues should be encouraged to think more widely and be creative! Having a nursing presence in service improvement projects, for instance, can have an impact on service design and delivery, and ultimately patient care.

Activity 8.6   Leadership and management

Make some time to sit down with a colleague and discuss their CPD goals. This may be someone who is new to your area, or someone you are buddying. Use Egan's model to understand what is important to them and define their goals. Capture the actions and make time to meet up to review them. After the meeting, reflect on your involvement and include this in your portfolio. Consider what went well, what you could have done differently and what you might change for your next meeting as a result of this learning.

There is no model answer as this activity is based upon your own experience.

Hopefully you will find that Activity 8.6 helps colleagues to formalise their CPD goals. This can directly link professional development activities to improving patient outcomes. It can be a particularly powerful way to motivate individuals, including those who lack confidence or are new to a clinical area.

Chapter summary

As a result of reading this chapter and completing the activities, you should clearly see the importance of resilience and mental wellbeing to the placement learning context and your developing supervisor/assessor role. Your skills as a practice supervisor/assessor can be developed by applying knowledge from everyday techniques (five ways to wellbeing) and more formal models (Egan's model and cognitive behavioural approaches). This chapter has highlighted that looking after our mental wellbeing can enhance our resilience and help us cope with the stresses associated with being a health professional and supervisor/assessor. This can be particularly useful in enabling us to *bounce back* from very difficult situations. The importance of CPD in improving confidence, competence, service delivery and care is highlighted – not only your own CPD but also through supporting others to engage in this activity.

Activity answers

Activity 8.3: Evidence-based practice and research (p167)

In relation to the Scenario, the activities that fit against the *five ways* are:

- connect – Tina talked with her colleagues;
- be active – Tina was going swimming;

- take notice – Daphne noticed how caring and compassionate Tina was;
- learn – Tina engaged in clinical supervision;
- give – Tina is a member of a journal club.

Activity 8.4: Critical thinking (p170)

	Applying the ABC to the Scenario	Further information
A = Activating event	In the Scenario this is the anaesthetist and surgeon complaining to the ward manager.	This can be something that we **directly** experience, as in David's case, or something we **observe**, e.g. a car crash.
B = Beliefs	David is worried that the error could be considered a *near miss* … He thinks people are now questioning his competence. He thinks he is an embarrassment to his profession.	**Beliefs** can also be termed **thoughts** or **cognitions**. The cognitive behavioural approach is based on evidence that **negative beliefs** or **thoughts** give rise to unpleasant physical feelings and **influence** our mood and behaviours.
C = Consequence First one is feelings (physical)	David has butterflies in his stomach when he thinks about a student engaging in pre-operative care.	There are three aspects to consequence: physical feelings, emotions and behaviours. These are outlined in the following rows of the table. Physical sensations can be very **unpleasant**, and people may think they are about to faint, etc.
C = Consequence Second one is feelings (emotional)	He feels embarrassed and ashamed.	**Distressing** emotions such as apprehension, anxiety and depression are **commonly reported**.
C = Consequence Third one is behaviour	David is now constantly double/triple checking that students have passed on all the information and does not allow them to *hand over* patient care anymore. Behaviours may be things individuals have stopped doing – such as allowing students to hand over, or started doing, e.g. double and triple checking student actions.	Behaviours are **usually observable** to others. However, they **may not** be. For example, someone might count in threes to help them **cope** with a stressful situation. Counting aloud can be observed by others, but counting in one's head cannot. However, they are both behaviours as they are **intentional** acts. The behaviours someone adopts may be a way of reducing the unpleasant physical sensations, e.g. one common **behavioural consequence** is **avoiding** a situation which someone finds stressful.

Further reading

Egan, G (2013) *The Skilled Helper: A Problem-Management and Opportunity-Development Approach to Helping*. Belmont, CA: Cengage Learning.

A great book if you want to find out more about this mentoring/helping model.

NHS Professionals (2019) *Your Health and Wellbeing Hub.* Available online at: **www. nhsprofessionals.nhs.uk/health-and-wellbeing**.

A comprehensive resource, specifically aimed at health professionals, that could be used for yourself, learners and colleagues.

Powell, T (2009) *The Mental Health Handbook, 3rd edition: A Cognitive Behavioural Approach.* London: Speechmark Publishing Ltd.

This is a very accessible handbook with activities and templates.

Useful websites

Health Education England: **www.hee.nhs.uk**.

Pages on advanced clinical practice, which includes information on the four pillars you may wish to assess your CPD needs against.

NMC: **www.nmc.org.uk**.

Pages with information on revalidation and the revalidation process. It includes a range of templates you can complete to provide evidence to support your revalidation.

Glossary

Approved Educational Institution (AEI) this is an educational institution, usually a university, that has been approved by the NMC to deliver NMC-approved programmes. In addition to the institution being approved, individual courses must also be approved (see **NMC-approved programme**).

autonomy in relation to nursing practice, this is linked to the ability to demonstrate competence by working independently and confidently making decisions, and exercising clinical reasoning and judgement.

Care Quality Commission (CQC) the independent regulator of health and adult social care in England. It has a number of standards that all health and social care services must meet. It regulates a wide range of services including hospitals, GP practices, dental practices, ambulance services, care homes and home-care agencies. The CQC monitors and inspects services to see whether they are safe, effective, caring, responsive and well led.

communities of practice (CoPs) a group of individuals who come together (face to face or online) to generate and share ideas and seek solutions to common problems. They may not regularly work together, but will be experiencing similar problems. CoPs are more effective when they are supported by organisations and employers while being allowed to create and innovate. They can be used in education to focus on areas such as assessment methods or ways to enhance distance learning. In practice, they may be used to innovate around options to hospital admission.

empowerment when individuals are given opportunities to work on issues that are important to them. They are seen as part of the solution and are encouraged to take control and make decisions.

experiential learning learning from experience. It has a structured approach that includes reflecting on and making sense of our experiences in order to make any necessary changes to improve our practice.

fitness to practise (FtP) a term used by the NMC. Being fit to practise requires a nurse or midwife to have the skills, knowledge, good health and good character to do their job safely and effectively. All registered nurses and midwives must follow the NMC Code. If an allegation is made to the NMC regarding a nurse or midwife's fitness to practise, it will investigate whether the registrant meets its standards for skills, education and behaviour. As a result, the NMC may remove an individual from the register permanently or for a set period of time.

formative assessment a type of assessment that can be used throughout a period of study. It gives individuals the opportunity to see how they are progressing and provides feedback on their performance to enable them to improve.

interprofessional learning a range of professionals learning *with, from and about* each other. There are shared learning opportunities including modules and practice learning.

mentoring and coaching often used interchangeably. Coaching is usually a short-term relationship focusing on specific goals or development areas. The coach may have expertise in an area the person wishes to develop. Mentoring is a longer-term relationship and has a less focused approach. It may be concerned with longer-term development and career planning.

multi-professional working more than one professional group working in an area such as a ward or community setting. There may be some sharing of tasks and responsibilities.

NMC-approved programme this is a course that has been approved by the NMC as meeting its standards and requirements. NMC-approved programmes enable people who have successfully completed them to be added to the NMC register or have their qualifications recorded on the NMC register. For example, a pre-registration nursing programme that, on successful completion, entitles someone to register as a nurse with the NMC.

NMC revalidation this was introduced by the NMC in April 2016 to replace PREP (post-registration education and practice). It is a process that occurs every three years and all NMC registrants must follow it to maintain their registration with the NMC.

Observed Structured Clinical Examination (OSCE) an assessment of clinical competence carried out in a structured and objective way. It is commonly used in pre-registration and postgraduate programmes. The OSCE format often comprises a number of assessment *stations* that students rotate around with various tasks to complete to assess competence. Stations may include history taking or using a clinical screening tool.

pedagogy concerned with the theory and practice of teaching. It is interested in how we learn and how that influences the way we teach.

Quality Assurance Agency (QAA) works across all four nations of the UK. It is the independent body entrusted with monitoring and advising on standards and quality in UK higher education. This includes the UK Quality Code for Higher Education.

reasonable adjustments measures put in places to ensure disabled students are enabled to achieve their full potential in both practice- and campus-based learning environments. These may include altered shift patterns or specialist equipment such as speech recognition software for students with dyslexia.

recognition of prior learning (RPL) a process used by AEIs that takes into account any previous learning undertaken by a student. This learning may have been formal learning carrying academic credit, such as a course. Or it may be less formal learning, for example someone who has undertaken an audit as part of their role. They can use this to evidence the necessary knowledge required for a module or course. RPL is often used as part of the entrance requirements for a course or to enable students to reduce the number of modules they need to study on a course.

self-efficacy   our confidence in succeeding in a given situation or to perform a task.

summative assessment   usually completed at the end of a period of study, such as a module or placement. Students are graded on the performance, either pass/fail or a specific grade, and this is used to determine their progression, final mark or grade or classification.

uni-professional   a single professional group, such as nursing or social work, often working in isolation from each other and with prescribed roles.

References

Aliakbari, F, Parvin, N, Heidari, M and Haghani, F (2015) Learning theories application in nursing education. Journal of Education and Health Promotion, 4. Available online at: www.ncbi.nlm.nih.gov/pmc/articles/PMC4355834.

Allen, S (2010) The revolution of nursing pedagogy: a transformational process. *Teaching and Learning in Nursing*, 5(1): 33–38.

Anonymous (2013) How can staff sickness rates be reduced in the NHS? *Nursing Times*, 109(13): 11.

Arnold, EC and Boggs, KU (2015) Interpersonal Relationships e-Book: Professional Communication Skills for Nurses. St Louis, MO: Elsevier Health Sciences.

Ashworth, G (2018) An alternative model for practice learning based on coaching. *Nursing Times*, 114(12): 30–32.

Askew, S and Lodge, C (2000) Gifts, ping-pong and loops: linking feedback and learning. In Askew, S (ed.) *Feedback for Learning*. London: Routledge.

Astrup, J (2018) The big story: raising standards for students. *Midwives Magazine*. Royal College of Midwives. Available online at: www.rcm.org.uk/news-views-and-analysis/news/the-big-story-raising-standards-for-students.

Atkins, J (2002) Interprofessional education today, yesterday and tomorrow. *Learning in Health and Social Care*, 1(3): 172–176.

Atkinson, S and Williams, P (2011) The involvement of service users in nursing students' education. *Learning Disability Practice (through 2013)*, 14(3): 18.

Austin, Z (2018) How to design and use learning objectives in clinical teaching. *Lung Cancer*, 15: 5.

Bandura, A (1977) *Social Learning Theory*. Englewood Cliffs, NJ: Prentice-Hall.

Boud, D (2015) Feedback: ensuring that it leads to enhanced learning. *The Clinical Teacher*, 12(1): 3–7.

Boud, D and Molloy, E (2013) Rethinking models of feedback for learning: the challenge of design. *Assessment & Evaluation in Higher Education*, 38(6): 698–712.

Boud, D, Cohen, R and Sampson, J (2014) *Peer Learning in Higher Education: Learning from and with Each Other*. Abingdon: Routledge.

Bozer, G and Jones, RJ (2018) Understanding the factors that determine workplace coaching effectiveness: a systematic literature review. *European Journal of Work and Organizational Psychology*, 27(3): 342–361.

Brooks, DC (2016) *ECAR Study of Undergraduate Students and Information Technology.* Available online at: https://er.educause.edu/~/media/files/library/2016/10/ers1605. pdf?la=en.

Brown, J, Morgan, A, Mason, J, Pope, N and Bosco, AM (2020) Student nurses' digital literacy levels: lessons for curricula. *Computers, Informatics, Nursing, 38*(9): 451–458.

Burton, J and Jackson, N (eds) (2003) *Work-Based Learning in Primary Care.* Abingdon: Radcliffe Publishing.

Caldwell, J, Dodd, K and Wilkes, C (2008) Developing a team mentoring model. *Nursing Standard, 23*(7): 35–39.

Carey, W, Philippon, DJ and Cummings, GG (2011) Coaching models for leadership development: an integrative review. *Journal of Leadership Studies, 5*(1), 51–69.

Carson-Stevens, A, Davies, MM, Jones, R, Chik, ADP, Robbé, IJ and Fiander, AN (2013) Framing patient consent for student involvement in pelvic examination: a dual model of autonomy. *Journal of Medical Ethics, 39*(11): 676–680.

Chandan, M and Watts, C (2012) Mentoring and pre-registration nurse education. Available online at: www.williscommission.org.uk/__data/assets/pdf_file/0009/479934/ Mentoring_and_preregistration_nurse_education.pdf.

Chapman, A (2017) Using the assessment process to overcome imposter syndrome in mature students. *Journal of Further and Higher Education, 41*(2): 112–119.

Christensen, M, Aubeeluck, A, Fergusson, D, Craft, J, Knight, J, Wirihana, L and Stupple, E (2016) Do student nurses experience imposter phenomenon? An international comparison of final year undergraduate nursing students' readiness for registration. *Journal of Advanced Nursing, 72*(11): 2784–2793.

Chuan, OL and Barnett, T (2012) Student, tutor and staff nurse perceptions of the clinical learning environment. *Nurse Education in Practice, 12*(4): 192–197.

Clarke, D, Williamson, GR and Kane, A (2018) Could students' experiences of clinical placements be enhanced by implementing a Collaborative Learning in Practice (CliP) model? *Nurse Education in Practice,* March: 1–3.

Cox, E, Bachkirova, T and Clutterbuck, DA (eds) (2014) *The Complete Handbook of Coaching.* London: Sage/Learning Matters.

Cummings, J and Bennett, V (2012) *Compassion in Practice.* NHS Commissioning Board, Department of Health.

Davies, HT and Nutley, SM (2000) Developing learning organisations in the new NHS. *BMJ: British Medical Journal, 320*(7240): 998.

Dean, E (2012) Building resilience. *Nursing Standard (through 2013), 26*(32): 16.

Department for Health and Human Services (2009) *Writing SMART Objectives.* Available online at: www.cdc.gov/healthyyouth/evaluation/pdf/brief3b.pdf.

Downey, M (2016) *Effective Modern Coaching: The Principles and Art of Successful Business Coaching.* London: LID Publishing.

Duffy, K (2003) Failing Students: A Qualitative Study of Factors That Influence the Decisions Regarding Assessment of Students' Competence in Practice. Glasgow: Caledonian Nursing and Midwifery Research Centre.

Duffy, K (2013) Providing constructive feedback to students during mentoring. *Nursing Standard (through 2013), 27*(31): 50.

Duffy, K (2015) Integrating the 6Cs of nursing into mentorship practice. *Nursing Standard (2014+), 29*(50): 49.

Duffy, K and Hardicre, J (2007a) Supporting failing students in practice. 1: Assessment. *Nursing Times, 103*(47): 28–29.

Duffy, K and Hardicre, J (2007b) Supporting failing students in practice. 2: Management. *Nursing Times, 103*(48): 28–29.

Egan, G (2013) The Skilled Helper: A Problem-Management and Opportunity-Development Approach to Helping. Belmont, CA: Cengage Learning.

Eick, SA, Williamson, GR and Heath, V (2012) A systematic review of placement-related attrition in nurse education. *International Journal of Nursing Studies, 49*(10): 1299–1309.

Eller, LS, Lev, EL and Feurer, A (2014) Key components of an effective mentoring relationship: a qualitative study. *Nurse Education Today, 34*(5): 815–820.

Elliott, T (2018) *Implementation of Collaborative Assessment & Learning Model (CALM): RCN Practice-Based Learning Innovations from around the UK.* Available online at: www.rcn.org.uk/professional-development/practice-based-learning/innovations-from-around-the-uk/implementation-of-collaborative-assessment-and-learning-model.

Ellis, P and Bach, S (2015) *Leadership, Management and Team Working in Nursing.* London: Sage/Learning Matters.

Evans, D and Brown, J (2017) Students in difficulty. In Cantillon, P, Wood, D and Yardley, S (eds) *ABC of Learning and Teaching in Medicine.* London: BMJ Books.

Fawcett, TJN and Rhynas, SJ (2014) Re-finding the 'human side' of human factors in nursing: helping student nurses to combine person-centred care with the rigours of patient safety. *Nurse Education Today, 34*(9): 1238–1241.

Felstead, IS and Springett, K (2016) An exploration of role model influence on adult nursing students' professional development: a phenomenological research study. *Nurse Education Today, 37*: 66–70.

Francis, R (2013) *Report of the Mid-Staffordshire NHS Foundation Trust Public Inquiry: Executive Summary (Vol. 947).* London: The Stationery Office. Available online at: http://webarchive.nationalarchives.gov.uk/20150407084231/www.midstaffspublicinquiry.com/report.

Gainsbury, S (2010) Nurse mentors still 'failing to fail' students. *Nursing Times, 106*(16): 2.

Gibbs, G (1988) Learning by Doing: A Guide to Teaching and Learning Methods. Oxford: Further Education Unit.

Glasper, A (2016) Moving from a blame culture to a learning culture in the NHS. *British Journal of Nursing*, *25*(7): 410–411.

Gravells, A (2017) *Principles and Practices of Teaching and Training: A Guide for Teachers and Trainers in the FE and Skills Sector*. London: Sage/Learning Matters.

Hallin, K (2014) Nursing students at a university: a study about learning style preferences. *Nurse Education Today*, *34*(12): 1443–1449.

Hamshire, C, Willgoss, TG and Wibberley, C (2012) 'The placement was probably the tipping point': the narratives of recently discontinued students. *Nurse Education in Practice*, *12*(4): 182–186.

Haraldseid, C, Friberg, F and Aase, K (2016) How can students contribute? A qualitative study of active student involvement in development of technological learning material for clinical skills training. *BMC Nursing*, *15*(1): 2.

Health and Safety Executive (n.d.) *Stress at Work*. Available online at: www.hse.gov.uk/stress/signs.htm.

Health Education England (n.d.) Alternative approaches to mentorship: an introduction to new models. Available online at: http://practiceassessor.bournemouth.ac.uk/assets/1512484653129_Alternative%20approaches%20to%20mentorship.docx.

Health Education England (2014) *Nurses Leaving Practice*. Available online at: www.hee.nhs.uk/sites/default/files/documents/Nurses%20leaving%20practice%20-%20Literature%20Review.pdf.

Health Education England (2015) *Managing Foundation Programme Doctors with Differing Needs*. Available online at: https://madeinheene.hee.nhs.uk/Portals/0/Policies/Foundation%20Specific/Managing%20FD%20different%20needs/Managing%20Foundation%20Programme%20Doctors%20with%20Differing%20Needs.pdf?ver=2016-05-31-134330-893.

Health Education England (2016) *Values-Based Recruitment Framework*. Available online at: www.hee.nhs.uk/our-work/values-based-recruitment.

Health Education England (2017a) *Multi-Professional Framework for Advanced Clinical Practice in England*. Available online at: www.hee.nhs.uk/sites/default/files/documents/multi-professionalframeworkforadvancedclinicalpracticeinengland.pdf.

Health Education England (2017b) *Case Study: Implementing Collaborative Learning in Practice – A New Way of Learning for Nursing Students*. Workforce Information Network. Available online at: https://healthacademy.lancsteachinghospitals.nhs.uk/download/doc/docm93jijm4n4874.pdf?ver=9427.

Health Education England (2018) *HEE Diversity and Inclusion: Our Strategic Framework 2018–2022*. Available online at: www.hee.nhs.uk/sites/default/files/documents/Diversity%20and%20Inclusion%20-%20Our%20Strategic%20Framework.pdf.

Health Education England (2019) *The Topol Review: Preparing the Healthcare Workforce to Deliver the Digital Future*. Available online at: https://topol.hee.nhs.uk.

Helminen, K, Tossavainen, K and Turunen, H (2014) Assessing clinical practice of student nurses: views of teachers, mentors and students. Nurse Education Today, 34(8): 1161–1166.

Helminen, K, Coco, K, Johnson, M, Turunen, H and Tossavainen, K (2016) Summative assessment of clinical practice of student nurses: a review of the literature. *International Journal of Nursing Studies, 53*: 308–319.

Honey, P and Mumford, A (2000) *The Learning Styles Helper's Guide*. Maidenhead: Peter Honey Publications.

Howatson-Jones, L (2016) *Reflective Practice in Nursing*. London: Sage/Learning Matters.

Hughes, LJ, Mitchell, M and Johnston, AN (2016) 'Failure to fail' in nursing: a catch phrase or a real issue? A systematic integrative literature review. *Nurse Education in Practice, 20*: 54–63.

Hunt, LA, McGee, P, Gutteridge, R and Hughes, M (2016) Manipulating mentors' assessment decisions: do underperforming student nurses use coercive strategies to influence mentors' practical assessment decisions? *Nurse Education in Practice, 20*: 154–162.

Huybrecht, S, Loeckx, W, Quaeyhaegens, Y, De Tobel, D and Mistiaen, W (2011) Mentoring in nursing education: perceived characteristics of mentors and the consequences of mentorship. *Nurse Education Today, 31*(3): 274–278.

Jack, K, Hamshire, C and Chambers, A (2017) The influence of role models in undergraduate nurse education. *Journal of Clinical Nursing, 26*(23–24): 4707–4715.

Jackson, PZ and McKergow, M (2006) *The Solutions Focus: Making Coaching and Change SIMPLE*. Boston, MA: Nicholas Brealey Publishing, 2nd edition.

Jarrett, C (2010) Feeling like a fraud. *Psychologist, 23*(5): 380–383.

Jervis, A and Tilki, M (2011) Why are nurse mentors failing to fail student nurses who do not meet clinical performance standards? *British Journal of Nursing, 20*(9): 582–587.

Jones, K, Warren, A and Davies, A (2015) Mind the Gap: Exploring the Needs of Early Career Nurses and Midwives in the Workplace. Birmingham: Health Education England.

Kelton, MF (2014) Clinical coaching: an innovative role to improve marginal nursing students' clinical practice. *Nurse Education in Practice, 14*(6): 709–713.

Kemper, KJ, Mo, X and Khayat, R (2015) Are mindfulness and self-compassion associated with sleep and resilience in health professionals? *The Journal of Alternative and Complementary Medicine, 21*(8): 496–503.

Keogh, B (2013) *Review into the Quality of Care and Treatment Provided by 14 Hospital Trusts in England: Overview Report*. NHS England. Available online at: www.nhs.uk/NHSEngland/bruce-keogh-review/Documents/outcomes/keogh-review-final-report.pdf.

Kirkwood, TB, Bond, J, May, C, McKeith, I and Teh, MM (2014) Foresight mental capital and wellbeing project: mental capital through life – future challenges. In Chen, PY and Cooper, C (eds) *Wellbeing: A Complete Reference Guide*. New York: Wiley, pp1–90.

Knowles, MS (1968) Andragogy, not pedagogy. *Adult Leadership, 16*(10): 350–352.

Knowles, MS (1980) *The Modern Practice of Adult Education: From Pedagogy to Andragogy*. Chicago, IL: Follet Publishing, Association Press.

Koen, MP, Van Eeden, C and Wissing, MP (2011) The prevalence of resilience in a group of professional nurses. *Health SA Gesondheid (Online), 16*(1): 1–11. Available online at: https://hsag.co.za/index.php/hsag/article/view/576.

Kolb, DA (1984) *Experiential Learning: Experience as the Source of Learning and Development.* Englewood Cliffs, NJ: Prentice Hall.

Lancashire Teaching Hospitals (LTHT) (2017) *Case Study: Implementing Collaborative Learning in Practice – A New Way of Learning for Nursing Students.* Available online at: www.ewin.nhs.uk/sites/default/files/eWIN%20Case%20Study%20-%20CLIP%20-%20a%20new%20way%20of%20learning%20for%20student%20nurses.pdf.

Lave, J and Wenger, E (1991) *Situated Learning: Legitimate Peripheral Participation.* Cambridge: Cambridge University Press.

Lawson, L (2010) Supporting Mentors and Clinical Educators: A Collaborative Project into the Development of Knowledge and Skills to Enhance Clinical Education Practice. University of Hertfordshire, unpublished report.

L'Ecuyer, KM (2019) Clinical education of nursing students with learning difficulties: an integrative review (part 1). *Nurse Education in Practice, 34*: 173–184.

Lestander, Ö, Lehto, N and Engström, Å (2016) Nursing students' perceptions of learning after high fidelity simulation: effects of a three-step post-simulation reflection model. *Nurse Education Today, 40*: 219–224.

Lewin (2007) Clinical learning environments for student nurses: key indices from two studies compared over a 25-year period. *Nurse Education in Practice, 7*: 238–246.

Lobo, C, Arthur, A and Lattimer, V (2014) *Collaborative Learning in Practice (CLiP) for Pre-Registration Nursing Students.* Health Education England, University of East Anglia. Available online at: www.charleneloboconsulting.com/wp-content/uploads/CLiP-Paper-final-version-Sept-14.pdf.

MacIntosh, T (2015) The link lecturer role: inconsistent and incongruent realities. *Nurse Education Today, 35*(3): e8–e13.

Maslow, AH (1943) A theory of human motivation. *Psychological Review, 50*(4): 370–396.

McDermid, F, Peters, K, Daly, J and Jackson, D (2016) Developing resilience: stories from novice nurse academics. *Nurse Education Today, 38*: 29–35.

McDonald, S and Ahern, K (2002) Physical and emotional effects of whistle blowing. *Journal of Psychosocial Nursing and Mental Health Services, 40*(1): 14–27.

McDonough, K (2016) How to teach interprofessional learners. In Mookherjee, S and Cosgrove, E (eds) *Handbook of Clinical Teaching.* Cham: Springer.

McKellar, L and Graham, K (2017) A review of the literature to inform a best-practice clinical supervision model for midwifery students in Australia. *Nurse Education in Practice, 24*: 92–98.

Mitchell, G. (2019) Trusts called on to do more to support stressed nursing staff. *Nursing Times.* Available online at: www.nursingtimes.net/news/workforce/trusts-called-on-to-do-more-to-support-stressed-nursing-staff-05-04-2019.

National Nursing Research Unit (2009) Nursing competence: what are we assessing and how should it be measured? *Policy.* Issue 18. King's College London. Available online at: www.kcl.ac.uk/nursing/research/nnru/policy/Policy-Plus-Issues-by-Theme/Boundaries-regulation-competence/PolicyIssue18.pdf.

Neenan, M and Dryden, W (2013) *Life Coaching: A Cognitive Behavioural Approach.* London: Routledge.

Newnham-Kanas, C, Morrow, D and Irwin, JD (2010) Motivational coaching: a functional juxtaposition of three methods for health behaviour change – motivational interviewing, coaching, and skilled helping. *International Journal of Evidence-Based Coaching & Mentoring,* 8(2): 27–48.

NHS Choices (2017) *Moodzone: How to Deal with Stress.* Available online at: www.nhs.uk/conditions/stress-anxiety-depression/understanding-stress.

NHS Employers (2017) *Multigenerational Workforce.* Available online at: www.nhsemployers.org/your-workforce/plan/recruiting-from-your-community/engaging-with-and-recruiting-from-across-your-local-community/multigenerational-workforce.

NHS Employers (2020) *How to Embed Flexible Working for Nurses.* Available online at: www.nhsemployers.org/-/media/Employers/Publications/Workforce-Supply/Retention/NHSE—Flexible-Working-Guidebook.pdf.

NHS England (2014) *Five Year Forward View.* Available online at: www.england.nhs.uk/wp-content/uploads/2014/10/5yfv-web.pdf.

NHS England (2015) The NHS Constitution. *The NHS Belongs to Us All.* London: NHS England.

NHS England (2019) *The NHS Long Term Plan.* London: NHS England. Available online at: www.longtermplan.nhs.uk/publication/nhs-long-term-plan.

NHS Executive (2015) New 'duty of candour' guidance published for NHS staff. *Workforce and Training News.* Available online at: www.nationalhealthexecutive.com/Health-Care-News/new-duty-of-candour-guidance-published-for-nhs-staff.

NHS Improvement (2018) *Active Listening.* Available online at: https://improvement.nhs.uk/resources/active-listening.

Nursing and Midwifery Council (NMC) (n.d.) *Professional Duty of Candour Guidance.* Available online at: www.nmc.org.uk/standards/guidance/the-professional-duty-of-candour/read-the-professional-duty-of-candour.

Nursing and Midwifery Council (NMC) (2008) Standards to Support Learning and Assessment in Practice: NMC Standards for Mentors, Practice Teachers and Teachers. London: Nursing and Midwifery Council.

Nursing and Midwifery Council (NMC) (2010) *Standards for Pre-Registration Nursing Education.* London: Nursing and Midwifery Council.

Nursing and Midwifery Council (NMC) (2011) *Standards for Competence for Registered Midwives.* London: Nursing and Midwifery Council. Available online at: www.nmc.org.uk/globalassets/sitedocuments/standards/nmc-standards-for-competence-for-registered-midwives.pdf.

Nursing and Midwifery Council (NMC) (2015) *The Code: Professional Standards of Practice and Behaviour for Nurses and Midwives.* London: Nursing and Midwifery Council. Available online at: www.nmc.org.uk/globalassets/sitedocuments/nmc-publications/nmc-code.pdf.

Nursing and Midwifery Council (NMC) (2017a) *How to Revalidate with the NMC: Requirements for Renewing Your Registration.* Available online at: www.nmc.org.uk/globalassets/sitedocuments/revalidation/how-to-revalidate-booklet.pdf.

Nursing and Midwifery Council (NMC) (2017b) *Enabling Professionalism in Nursing and Midwifery Practice.* London: Nursing and Midwifery Council. Available online at: www.nmc.org.uk/globalassets/sitedocuments/other-publications/enabling-professionalism.pdf.

Nursing and Midwifery Council (NMC) (2017c) *Raising Concerns: Guidance for Nurses and Midwives.* London: Nursing and Midwifery Council.

Nursing and Midwifery Council (NMC) (2018a) *Future Nurse: Standards of Proficiency for Registered Nurses.* London: Nursing and Midwifery Council. Available online at: www.nmc.org.uk/globalassets/sitedocuments/education-standards/future-nurse-proficiencies.pdf.

Nursing and Midwifery Council (NMC) (2018b) *Part 2: Standards for Student Supervision and Assessment.* London: Nursing and Midwifery Council. Available online at: www.nmc.org.uk/globalassets/sitedocuments/education-standards/student-supervision-assessment.pdf.

Nursing and Midwifery Council (NMC) (2018c) Meeting of the Council (March), Council Papers. Available online at: https://slidelegend.com/council-papers-march-2018-nmc_5ae35e147f8b9a18998b45a4.html.

Nursing and Midwifery Council (NMC) (2018d) Standards Framework for Nursing and Midwifery Education. Part 1 of Realising Professionalism: Standards for Education and Training. London: Nursing and Midwifery Council. Available online at: www.nmc.org.uk/standards-for-education-and-training/standards-framework-for-nursing-and-midwifery-education.

Nursing and Midwifery Council (NMC) (2018e) *Standards of Proficiency for Nursing Associates.* London: Nursing and Midwifery Council.

Nursing and Midwifery Council (NMC) (2019a) *Reasonable Adjustments (If Applicable) Guidance.* London: Nursing and Midwifery Council. Available online at: www.nmc.org.uk/supporting-information-on-standards-for-student-supervision-and-assessment/student-empowerment/what-to-expect/reasonable-adjustments-if-applicable.

Nursing and Midwifery Council (NMC) (2019b) *Standards of Proficiency for Midwives.* London: Nursing and Midwifery Council.

Nursing and Midwifery Council (NMC) (2021) *Recovery and Emergency Programme Standards.* London: Nursing and Midwifery Council. Available online at: www.nmc.org.uk/standards-for-education-and-training/emergency-education-standards.

Office for National Statistics (2019) *Exploring the UK's Digital Divide.* Available online at: www.ons.gov.uk/peoplepopulationandcommunity/householdcharacteristics/homeinternetandsocialmediausage.

Olson, MH (2015) *Introduction to Theories of Learning.* New York: Routledge.

Palmer, S (2008) The PRACTICE model of coaching: towards a solution-focused approach. *Coaching Psychology International, 1*(1): 4–8.

Pålsson, Y, Mårtensson, G, Swenne, CL, Ädel, E and Engström, M (2017) A peer learning intervention for nursing students in clinical practice education: a quasi-experimental study. *Nurse Education Today, 51*: 81–87.

Perry, C, Henderson, A and Grealish, L (2018) The behaviours of nurses that increase student accountability for learning in clinical practice: an integrative review. *Nurse Education Today, 65*: 177–186.

Piggot-Irvine, E and Biggs, K (2020) *Leadership Coaching, Mentoring, Counselling or Supervision? One Way Is Not Enough.* Cambridge: Cambridge Scholars Publishing.

Pollock, CHF, Rice, AM and McMillan, A (2015) Mentors' and students' perspectives on feedback in practice assessment: a literature review. *NHS Education for Scotland.* Available online at: www.nes.scot.nhs.uk/media/3288312/mentors_and_students_perspectives_on_feedback_in_practice_assessment.pdf.

Powell, T (2009) The Mental Health Handbook, 3rd edition: A Cognitive Behavioural Approach. London: Speechmark Publishing Ltd.

Pritchard, E and Gidman, J (2012) Effective mentoring in the community setting. *British Journal of Community Nursing, 17*(3): 119–124.

Robinson, S, Cornish, J, Driscoll, C, Knutton, S, Corben, V and Stevenson, T (2012) *Sustaining and Managing the Delivery of Student Nurse Mentorship: Roles, Resources, Standards, and Debates.* Report for NHS London 'Readiness for Work' programme. National Nursing Research Unit, King's College London. Available online at: www.kcl.ac.uk/nursing/research/.../Nurse-Mentorship-Short-Report-Nov12.pdf.

Rosser, E (2017) Education does matter: nursing apprenticeships in the workforce. *British Journal of Nursing, 26*(7): 434.

Royal College of Nursing (RCN) (n.d.) *Patient Safety and Human Factors.* Available online at: www.rcn.org.uk/clinical-topics/patient-safety-and-human-factors.

Royal College of Nursing (RCN) (2007) Guidance for Mentors of Nursing Students and Midwives: An RCN Toolkit. London: RCN.

Royal College of Nursing (RCN) (2016a) *RCN Factsheet: Continuing Professional Development (CPD) for Nurses Working in the United Kingdom (UK).* Available online at: www.rcn.org.uk/about-us/policy-briefings/pol-1614.

Royal College of Nursing (RCN) (2016b) *RCN Mentorship Project 2015: From Today's Support in Practice to Tomorrow's Vision for Excellence.* Rapid Evidence Review. London: RCN.

Royal College of Nursing (RCN) (2017a) *Helping Students Get the Best from Their Practice Placements: A Royal College of Nursing Toolkit.* Available online at: file://staffhome.hallam.shu.ac.uk/STAFFHOME1/l/hscjl/MyWork/Jos%20stuff/send%20to%20Julie/PUB-006035.pdf.

Royal College of Nursing (RCN) (2017b) Response to NMC Consultation Document on: Standards of Proficiency for Registered Nurses; Education Framework; Standards for Education and Training; Prescribing and Standards for Medicines Management. Available online at: www.rcn.org.uk/-/media/royal-college-of-nursing/…/2017/…/pdf-006447.pdf.

Royal College of Nursing (RCN) (2017c) *Reasonable Adjustments: The Peer Support Service Guide for Members Affected by Disability in the Workplace.* Available online at: www.rcn.org.uk/professional-development/publications/pub-006595.

Scott, SV (2014) Practising what we preach: towards a student-centred definition of feedback. *Teaching in Higher Education, 19*(1): 49–57.

Scottish Social Services Council (2016) *Coaching Learning Resource.* Available online at: www.stepintoleadership.info/assets/pdf/SSSC%20Coaching%20Aug%2016%20master.pdf.

Seymour-Walsh, A (2016) Addressing clinician burnout: how can we build resilience in tomorrow's health professionals? *Resuscitation, 106*: e48–e49.

Sonnak, C and Towell, T (2001) The impostor phenomenon in British university students: relationships between self-esteem, mental health, parental rearing style and socioeconomic status. *Personality and Individual Differences, 31*(6): 863–874.

Su, WM and Osisek, PJ (2011) The revised Bloom's Taxonomy: implications for educating nurses. *The Journal of Continuing Education in Nursing, 42*(7): 321–327.

Tasselli, S (2015) Social networks and inter-professional knowledge transfer: the case of healthcare professionals. *Organization Studies, 36*(7): 841–872.

Taylor, DCM and Hamdy, H (2013) Adult learning theories: implications for learning and teaching in medical education: AMEE Guide No. 83. *Medical Teacher, 35*(11): e1561–e1572.

Tee, SR, Owens, K, Plowright, S, Ramnath, P, Rourke, S, James, C and Bayliss, J (2010) Being reasonable: supporting disabled nursing students in practice. *Nurse Education in Practice, 10*(4): 216–221.

The Institute for Innovation and Improvement (2010) *SBAR Communication Tool: Situation, Background, Assessment, Recommendation.* Available online at: www.england.nhs.uk/improvement-hub/wp-content/uploads/sites/44/2017/11/SBAR-Implementation-and-Training-Guide.pdf.

Vinales, JJ (2015) Exploring failure to fail in pre-registration nursing. *British Journal of Nursing, 24*(5): 284–288.

Whitelock, D, Thorpe, M and Galley, R (2015) Student workload: a case study of its significance, evaluation and management at the Open University. *Distance Education, 36*(2): 161–176.

Whitmore, J. (2017) *Coaching for Performance: The Principles and Practice of Coaching and Leadership, 5th edition.* Boston, MA: N. Brealey Publishing.

Willingham, DT, Hughes, EM and Dobolyi, DG (2015) The scientific status of learning styles theories. *Teaching of Psychology, 42*(3): 266–271.

Willis Commission (2012) *Quality with Compassion: The Future of Nursing Education.* Available online at: www.williscommission.org.uk/__data/assets/pdf_file/0007/495115/Willis_commission_report_Jan_2013.pdf.

Willis, P and Shape of Caring Review (2015) Raising the Bar: Shape of Caring – A Review of the Future Education and Training of Registered Nurses and Care Assistants. London: Health Education England.

World Health Organization (2013) *Interprofessional Collaborative Practice in Primary Health Care: Nursing and Midwifery Perspectives – Six Case Studies.* Available online at: www.who.int/hrh/resources/IPE_SixCaseStudies.pdf.

Wosinski, J, Belcher, AE, Dürrenberger, Y, Allin, AC, Stormacq, C and Gerson, L (2018) Facilitating problem-based learning among undergraduate nursing students: a qualitative systematic review. *Nurse Education Today, 60*: 67–74.

Index

Locators in **bold** refer to tables and those in *italics* to figures.